LIFE WITH A

BATTERY-OPERATED BRAIN:

A PATIENT'S GUIDE TO

DEEP BRAIN STIMULATION SURGERY

FOR PARKINSON'S DISEASE

LIFE WITH A
BATTERY-OPERATED BRAIN:

A PATIENT'S GUIDE TO
DEEP BRAIN STIMULATION SURGERY
FOR PARKINSON'S DISEASE

JACKIE HUNT CHRISTENSEN

AUTHOR OF *THE FIRST YEAR: PARKINSON'S DISEASE,
AN ESSENTIAL GUIDE FOR THE NEWLY DIAGNOSED*

LANGDON STREET PRESS
MINNEAPOLIS, MINNESOTA

Langdon Street Press
212 3ʳᵈ Avenue North, Suite 290
Minneapolis, MN 55401
612.455.2293
www.langdonstreetpress.com

ISBN - 978-1-934938-26-3
ISBN - 1-934938-26-2
LCCN - 2009922269

Book sales for North America and international:
Itasca Books, 3501 Highway 100 South, Suite 220
Minneapolis, MN 55416
Phone: 952.345.4488 (toll free 1.800.901.3480)
Fax: 952.920.0541; email to orders@itascabooks.com

Cover Design by Sophie Chi
Typeset by Kristeen Wegner

Printed in the United States of America

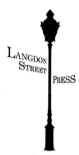

L ANGDON
S TREET
PRESS

For my father, who deserves to be reincarnated as an Olympic athlete!

TABLE OF CONTENTS

Introduction

I remember being at the Cleveland Clinic in October 2005. My book, *The First Year: Parkinson's Disease, an Essential Guide for the Newly Diagnosed*, had just been published by Marlowe and Company, and I was very excited. When I mentioned it to Sierra Farris, a certified physician's assistant (PA-C) and programmer, as she was conducting part of my evaluation for deep brain stimulation (DBS) surgery, she said, "You know what you should write about? DBS." Her point was that there were no books available that had straightforward information for patients about the surgical procedures and life afterward.

I thought about the information I had seen on DBS. Other than the Medtronic DVD about the Activa neurostimulator system, there wasn't really anything, except some newsletter articles by the various Parkinson's disease (PD) groups. I then checked online. In December 2005, there was one book available, and that was a medical textbook that cost $195. Because there is such a lack of information for people who are contemplating DBS or who have already had surgery, I decided that it might be worthwhile to provide information about that experience. Just as I had never dreamed that I would write one book, I had not made plans to write another.

My goal with this book is to provide you—as someone who has PD, as a caregiver to someone with the disease, or as a clinician who treats Parkinson's patients—with as much information as possible about DBS.

You can use this newfound knowledge to inform your decision to consider surgery or to learn more about what post-op life can be like.

To make the material more "digestible" and, I hope, a little more interesting, I will use excerpts from the blog that I began keeping before my surgery, personal experiences, and anecdotes from other people who have had DBS surgery.

Disclaimer: Please note that this book is not intended to dispense medical advice. Any decisions you make should be in consultation with your own physician or health-care professional.

Although DBS has been used for years to treat essential tremor and is now being tried as a therapy for depression, obsessive-compulsive disorder (OCD), Tourette's syndrome, and other conditions, I will be writing mainly from my perspective of someone with Parkinson's (or "Parkies," as I prefer to call those of us who live with the disease. I find it less pretentious than the other commonly used term, "Parkinsonian.") I have written this book without the involvement of Medtronic, maker of the Soletra system that is implanted in my body.

Chapter One
What Is Deep Brain Stimulation?

Note: Sierra Farris contributed to this chapter. She is a certified physician's assistant (PA-C) who has been a DBS programmer at Cleveland Clinic's Center for Neurological Restoration and at the Booth Gardner Parkinson Center in Kirkland, Washington.

You may have heard people speak in hushed, awed tones about "the surgery" that is performed around the country and around the world to treat many of the symptoms of **essential tremor** (ET), **Parkinson's disease** (PD), and **dystonia**. (Some people with PD also have ET; dystonia is also common in PD patients.) This "surgery" is called deep brain stimulation (DBS). It has also been used experimentally to treat depression, obsessive-compulsive disorder (OCD), Tourette's syndrome, and other neurological conditions.

Why anyone would say "Let's stick wires into someone's brain, run voltage through it, and see what happens!" is a mystery to me, but I guess that I should be glad that there are folks who think that way. Deep brain stimulation was first developed by Dr. Alim-Louis Benabid in the 1980s as alternatives to **pallidotomy** or **thalamotomy** surgeries. Those procedures make permanent lesions on the brain to control the movements associated with PD. Dr. Benabid published a paper on the first use of DBS in 1987 (Friehs, 2006).

Dr. Benabid worked with Medtronic, Inc., a medical device company in Minnesota, to commercially develop the system. The first clinical trials of the device began in 1992, and it became commercially available to treat tremor in Parkinson's disease and essential tremor in Europe, Canada, and Australia (Medtronic, 2008). Eventually, the technology made its way "across the pond" to America. It was used as an experimental therapy in the United States until 1997, when the Food and Drug Administration (FDA) approved it for treating essential tremor and tremor in Parkinson's disease. DBS received FDA approval for treatment of the **motor symptoms** (**dyskinesia**—a form of dystonia—muscle rigidity, and tremor) of advanced PD in January 2002.

Deep brain stimulation involves a surgical procedure in which one or two insulated electrical wires called "DBS **leads**" are put into parts of the brain where some of the symptoms of the particular condition originate. In Parkinson's disease, those areas are generally the **subthalamic nucleus** (STN) or the **globus pallidus interna** (GPi). Usually, two leads are used, because PD generally affects both sides of the body. When electrodes are placed in both sides of the brain, it is called **bilateral stimulation**. When treating ET, one lead inserted into the thalamus is typically used. This is called **unilateral stimulation.**

Many patients who have symptoms predominantly on one side have unilateral stimulation surgery. The other side can almost always be done later.

Choosing a DBS system is nothing like choosing a car or a stereo. As I write this, I know of only two companies who make the systems: Medtronic, Inc., and Advanced Neuromodulation Systems (ANS). Both have models for unilateral and bilateral stimulation. As of summer 2008, most surgeons use products from one company or the other but not both. If you require bilateral surgery, some neurosurgeons will ask you if you have a preference for one neurostimulator or two, or not. However, not all surgeons ask as a matter of course. During your evaluation, you might want to ask whether you have a choice in the matter.

COMPONENTS OF THE HARDWARE SYSTEM

A system consists of three parts:
1. An energy source. This is the **neurostimulator,** which also may be referred to as a "battery," "pacemaker," or implanted pulse generator (IPG). For the sake of consistency, I will refer to it as the "neurostimulator" throughout the book.
2. The lead wire (that's "lead" as in "to steer or direct," not the heavy metal). The tip of the lead that is inserted into the brain usually has four **electrodes**.
3. **Extension wire(s)** to connect them.

The neurostimulator is a bit smaller than a deck of playing cards. It is generally placed in the upper chest, but occasionally, the **neurosurgeon** may insert it into the abdomen for various reasons. For example, patients who shoot rifles or play hand bells may request abdominal placement, as this would allow them to continue to enjoy such a sport or hobby.

The neurostimulator is connected via an extension wire to the lead wire, deep inside the brain. The extension wire has prongs on one end that fit into the battery, with a connector on the other end. The lead wire, which is about the diameter of a piece of spaghetti, attaches to the extension wire by sliding into the connector and is secured with tiny screws. You may feel a bump behind the ear or somewhere around the upper neck area. That is the connector, where both wires come together. The lead wire continues from behind the ear to the top of the head, toward the front of the hairline.

There, you will find a plastic covering that is designed to avoid any movement of the lead wire, once it is placed into the brain. These coverings form the bumps that look like small horns about to burst from the head. The wires reach the brain through dime-sized holes that are drilled in the skull.

Once in the brain, the wire travels to the subthalamic nucleus (STN) or the globus pallidus (GPi) for PD or to the thalamus for PD and tremor.

All of this hardware is under the skin, by the way, so that you do not look like one of the Borg from TV's *Star Trek: The Next Generation*!

MORE ABOUT THE WIRES AND ELECTRODES

The wires in the DBS system are coated with a silicone material. This coating is pretty tough, but it is important to keep it that way. This is why people with DBS are discouraged from using spas, whirlpools, hot tubs, or saunas—the silicone could get too hot and melt! It may seem silly, but the engineers who designed the system issue warnings with good reason. If the silicone is breached, stimulation can leak out and cause symptoms, including tingling, crawling, muscle spasm, or shocks.

These wires come in different lengths. This is important because of height and proportion differences among patients and because, sometimes, the neurostimulator is placed in the belly area. I have met people with wires that are too short. Many of them report mild discomfort or a pulling sensation in their neck or head. Wires that are not the correct length also increase the risk of wire breakage.

Programmer Sierra Farris, PA-C, offers more of an explanation about the system components.

"In my experience, the longer the wire, the greater the potential for problems. I have no formal data to suggest that putting neurostimulator battery in the belly is not a good idea, but I have seen a few patients along the way [who] may have been happier if the neurostimulator had been placed somewhere else.

On the end of the wire are four tiny electrodes stacked one on top of the other. They are numbered zero, one, two, and three. Each one is 1.5 millimeters long—about the size of a grain of rice. Each tiny electrode connects to a hair-thin wire that is inside the silicone covering. The "zero" electrode is the one deepest or closest to the most distant tip of the wire. The spacing between the electrodes indicates which lead wire model you have [in the Medtronic Activa system]. The Model 3387 lead has 1.5-mm spacing and spans 10.5 millimeters. The Model 3389 lead has 0.5mm spacing between each electrode and spans 7.5 millimeters.

One model is not better than the other. It is how they are used that counts. Let's use a lead wire placed in the STN as an example. The STN spans around 5 to 6 millimeters—about the size of a jelly bean—and we are hoping to stimulate an area that is estimated to be about the size of one electrode, which is as big as a grain of rice. This stimulation area is sometimes referred to as the "motor territory" of the area in which it is placed (STN or GPi or thalamus.) Either lead wire will work, as long as at least one of the electrodes is in the target near the motor territory. An experienced neurosurgeon can help to ensure that the lead wire hits that target."

Advanced Neuromodulation Systems, Inc. (ANS), a division of St. Jude Medical, has begun clinical trials of their Libra system at twelve sites around the country, with 134 participants to receive DBS as part of the study. ANS is seeking FDA approval for the safety and efficacy of their device.

> The main difference between the Medtronic systems ... and ANS's devices is that Medtronic's delivers a constant-voltage pulse, which allows the current to vary, depending on the impedance of the brain, while its competitor delivers constant current, allowing the voltage to vary. ANS's vice president for scientific affairs, Tracy Cameron, notes that most animal research has been done using constant-current stimulators and hypothesizes that this approach may be more in tune with the brain's physiology (Moore, 2006).

Because the company is in the midst of the approval process, their representatives were unable to answer my questions about why a patient would choose their system over Medtronic's. I think that is a valid question for both companies. Of course, who knows what design changes both companies may be developing behind the scenes as I write this!

In a June 20, 2008, phone interview, Jennifer Armstrong of ANS said that the company's goal is "to push patient options to the next level" and noted that competition in the industry would help to drive those choices.

Medtronic often calls its Activa therapy a "pacemaker for the brain" because the system provides constant electrical stimulation, just as cardiac pacemakers do.

The neurostimulator provides electrical impulses that are intended to block (or normalize, depending on whom you ask) the signals that my brain is currently sending to my muscles—the messages telling my body to be very stiff or to writhe and flail around.

Because the housing for the neurostimulator also contains the battery, this entire piece of the system is replaced (and upgraded, if improvements have been made in the type of system the patient has) when the battery needs replacing.

The system is programmed to address each person's individual symptoms. With Parkinson's disease, it primarily helps with tremors (which I rarely have), rigidity, and **bradykinesia** (slowed movements). It doesn't really help with balance.

The **programming** process and battery replacement are covered in detail in upcoming chapters.

Figure 1:

Various Parts of the Brain That May Be Targeted in DBS Surgery

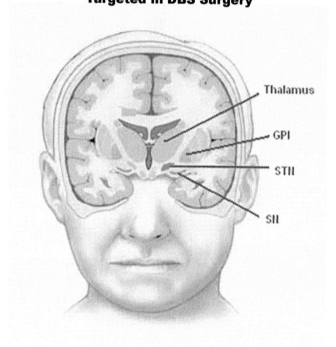

Source: (Colorado Neurological Institute, http://www.thecni.org/thompsoncenter/images/stn-dbs-illustration.jpg)

Chapter Two
Why Does DBS Work?

No one is completely certain how or why DBS works (Okun, Hernandez, and Foote)—that is a little scary. However, DBS does seem to work for the majority of qualified candidates if the wire is placed in the appropriate area of the brain.

The theory behind DBS goes something like this: when the brain is functioning normally, various parts of the brain send information to parts of the body and receive feedback. These messages tell our bodies when and how to move. With Parkinson's disease, the number and quality of messages going through the **dopamine system** is affected because of damage to neurons in the substantia nigra. DBS provides electrical stimuli to confuse or block the errant messages that tell your body to tremble or become stiff, which allows the correct instructions to get through. This "interference" helps to reduce tremors and rigidity, which facilitates faster movement.

Another way to look at it would be to imagine your brain as a large school. When functioning properly, the teachers teach the children all of the various subjects that the children need to know to be prepared for life in the real world. The children respond in class and do their homework—this shows that the information is getting through. But over time, a gang of rebellious kids forms. Sometimes they sit in their chairs and refuse to move. Other times, they do the "Hokey Pokey" when they are supposed to be writing homework. Soon, they affect all of the classrooms, so no one can learn anything. Finally, a teacher is hired specifically to deal with the troubled kids. No one knows whether it is due to respect or intimidation, but the new teacher's presence allows the other teachers to get back to the business of teaching. Every once in a while, the current students act up or another gang member moves in, but the school is more or less successful again.

The DBS system is a bit like that teacher—no one knows how long the teacher will be effective, but everyone enjoys the quiet atmosphere as long as it lasts.

Chapter Three
Making the Decision to
Be Evaluated for Surgery

To my mind, making the decision to investigate whether you are eligible for DBS has two stages: the internal discussion that you have with yourself, and the external discussion that you have with friends and family.

First, you decide that you are physically and emotionally ready to be evaluated. Finding this point might be likened to "hitting rock bottom" for someone with an addiction; each of us has our own level of misery that we can tolerate before we initiate change. I am convinced that this must be your own decision, not one you make for a loved one or to keep a job. Jobs and relationships end; Parkinson's doesn't, and DBS is meant to be a long-term solution.

I have met many other people living with PD who have said they had been too afraid to undergo the procedure or felt that their symptoms weren't "bad enough" yet. Unlike the motor symptoms of PD, which can be measured using standard procedures, an individual's fear of the surgery or willingness to tolerate symptoms cannot be measured.

I decided to do a survey, just to get a snapshot of how other people who have had DBS made their decisions to have surgery. I received fifty-eight responses, mostly from people with PD, although there were a few with ET or dystonia. It was not intended to be scientific in any way, but it does provide some interesting insights into the lives of fifty-eight people who have undergone deep brain stimulation surgery.

Here are some of the survey results that I find most compelling. (The entire survey is available in Appendix B.)

- Nearly 53 percent of respondents have had PD for more than twelve years.

- Nearly 42 percent were diagnosed with Parkinson's disease between the ages of 40 and 49. It is estimated that 15 percent of PD cases are diagnosed before age 40.

• Almost 33 percent pondered the decision to have DBS for one to three years before going through with the surgery.

• More than 18 percent of survey participants stated that they did not receive adequate information about DBS prior to undergoing the procedure.

• At least 65 percent of people surveyed said that they underwent DBS for themselves. Nearly 39 percent said that their doctors had recommended it. (Note that some people had more than one answer.)

• Sixty-three percent went to the surgeon or facility recommended by their doctors. More than 13 percent chose the surgeon/ facility based on their own research.

• When it came to the question of surgery-related pain, slightly more than half of respondents said that they had experienced pain (5.7 percent during surgery; 47.2 percent post-operatively).

• More than 73 percent of respondents said that they had no complications (infection, hemorrhage, etc.) with the surgery. At least 10 percent reportedly suffered infections.

• Most (87 percent) experienced at least one side effect. The most common side effect reported was a softer voice (58.9 percent), followed by slurred or garbled speech (38.9 percent), and decrease in balance abilities (37 percent).

When the surgery first became an option, researchers thought it was best to postpone it until all medication options had been tried and optimized. Now, there is an emerging school of thought that it might be more effective to do the surgery before symptoms are severe. In fact, clinical trials are enrolling participants to have DBS who have had PD for just a few years. Their disease progression will be tracked and compared to a similar group that receives medication only.

Meet with your neurologist to discuss the merits of being evaluated for the surgery now versus later.

If you are not currently seeing a **movement disorder specialist** or a neurologist who specializes in your condition, please do consult one. Professionals who treat your health problem on a frequent basis are much more likely to be aware of the most current research on DBS and other options. They are also more likely to have personal contacts with neurosurgeons that perform DBS.

The following is the first of several excerpts from my blog, titled "More Holes in My Head? My Journey toward Deep Brain Stimulation." (The blog is no longer available on-line.)

Deciding to have "the surgery"
Never say "Never"
Friday, December 23, 2005

Many of you know that DBS is something that I swore I would never ever do. For more than three years, I have endured well-meaning comments and letters—often from complete strangers!—asking if I had "heard about 'the surgery.'" I would thank them as politely as possible and think about the people I've known who have had DBS who have had a stroke or who had to be on intravenous antibiotics because of infections, or who had a surgeon who, when asked why the pacemakers were so close to the patient's collarbone, could not recall performing the operation! And I would think about folks whose speech had become slurred after the surgery. (The effects that PD has already had on my speech—making it softer and sometimes very halting, with little or no expression—are some of the symptoms that bothers me the most.)

But as I was doing research for my book and talked with more people who've had the operation, I found that even most of the people who've had what I would consider some major complications are still glad that they did it. That seemed like a pretty good testimonial.

Then there's the fact that I am taking a lot of medication around eight Sinemet1*** [levodopa] 25/100 tablets; plus a

---

1   *** Most of the people I know who have Parkinson's disease refer to the levodopa medication by its brand name, Sinemet, even if they take a generic version of the drug. I happen to have to take the brand name because the generics I have tried are not nearly as effective. For both of those reasons, I will use "Sinemet" throughout the book to refer to levodopa unless I am quoting another publication.

Sinemet CR; 100 mg of amantadine; 1–2 mg of Mirapex, an antidepressant; Ativan for anxiety and restless legs; and meds for my Crohn's disease) every day. I've been wondering what the long-term effects on my body might be from that extensive pharmacopeia.

And if the damn things worked consistently, I might not mind anyway, but lately, I have had considerable fluctuations in my "on" (meds working) time. The "off" time has gone from having my muscles decide that they will do their job very slowly, to a full-fledged sit-down strike. I have tried to express my willingness to negotiate a new "contract," but they are having none of it. So DBS will be sort of like "binding arbitration" for my brain.

Here are some of the reasons that others have undergone DBS surgery:

I did it so that I could play with my grandchildren.
~ Dawn, diagnosed with PD at age 42, DBS at age 54

I did it so as not to be a burden to my husband so soon.
~ Paulette, diagnosed with PD at age 45, DBS at age 61

I was young, in decent health, and wanted quality of life earlier rather than later.
~ Sean, diagnosed with PD in his 40s, DBS at 57

Some of my father's doctors really pushed for DBS (especially the ones with a financial benefit from performing DBS), while others said that because he was only 64 and doing fairly well, there was no rush to DBS but that it was certainly an option for future treatment. My father's medicines had been terribly mismanaged by his original Parkinson's doctor, who really preferred to handle MS patients. My father switched doctors and spent many months getting his medications back on track, to some measure of success. However, he still had a significant wearing-off effect and was taking pills (Sinemet, primarily) every two hours. Because of this, he/we began to seriously investigate DBS.
~ Anonymous caregiver

Once you have decided that *you* are ready, it is a good idea to talk with your care partner (if you have one), family, and friends about your decision. You will need their help and emotional support if you have the surgery, and you will need it if you are turned down for the procedure.

It really helped our family to sit down together and watch Medtronic's DVD, which explains the procedures. We discussed my younger son's concerns about the risks of surgery and about long-term complications. We also talked about the fact that the status quo clearly was not working and that was why I wanted to be evaluated for DBS.

Next, talk about expectations. You can avoid relationship "train wrecks" if you discuss everyone's expectations before you have the surgery. If possible, bring your neurologist or neurosurgeon into this discussion. He or she will let you know whether your expectations are realistic.

Paulette, 61, agreed that being "on the same page" as your family is important. She said, "Make sure that your family understands that it is not a cure. … My relatives just plain don't get it. My own mother (81 years old—may have something to do with it) thinks I can do anything, anytime."

Chapter Four
Work, DBS, and Disability/Social Security

People seek DBS at different ages, physical conditions, and states of employment. When I decided to be evaluated, I had already been on long-term disability for more than a year. Despite improvements in many of my physical symptoms, I am unable to work because of mental fatigue and problems with multitasking and executive function. Therefore, I have no experience with getting time off from work to have surgery, continuing employment after DBS, or returning to the workplace after time on disability.

I have spoken with others who have been through some of these circumstances, and there seem to be a few good recommendations:

- Do not return to work without permission from your doctor, particularly if you have been out of the workforce for a while.

- Do not expect to be able to do the same amount and type of work as you did before you were diagnosed with PD!

- If you have short-term or long-term disability insurance, review your policy to see when and if it comes into play with the surgery. Also, if you have not been working prior to surgery and have been collecting insurance benefits, ask how returning to work would affect the policy. For example, what happens to the benefits if you are able to return to *a* job, but not *the* job you'd had before.

- Go slowly. Give yourself time to heal. DBS is brain surgery, after all.

The "Ticket to Work" Program

The Social Security Administration, which administers social security and disability benefits, has a program called "Ticket to Work."

Special rules make it possible for people receiving social security disability benefits or supplemental security income (SSI) to work and still receive monthly payments.

And if you cannot continue working because of your medical condition, your benefits can start again—you may not have to file a new application.

Work incentives include:

- Continued cash benefits for a time while you work
- Continued Medicare or Medicaid while you work
- Help with education, training, and rehabilitation to start a new line of work

Source: *Working While Disabled—How We Can Help*
SSA Publication No. 05-10095, January 2008, ICN 468625

You can get a copy of this booklet online at http://www.ssa.gov/pubs/10095.html or by calling 1-800-772-1213 (TTY number, 1-800-325-0778) between 7 a.m. and 7 p.m. Eastern, Monday through Friday.

Chapter Five
The Evaluation Process

So, you are ready to be evaluated. Generally, neurologists will not recommend going through the evaluation process if they don't think that you are at least a fair candidate for surgery, but sometimes issues arise. Be aware that this can be a very anxious, stressful time, which will probably make your symptoms worse.

Are you a good candidate for evaluation for surgery? If you are a person living with Parkinson's disease, you are probably a good candidate for DBS if:

> • You have a diagnosis of idiopathic Parkinson's disease. This means that the cause is unknown, as opposed to familial PD or medication-induced PD. People who have been diagnosed with other forms of parkinsonism, such as multiple system atrophy (MSA), progressive supranuclear palsy (PSP), or Lewy Body disease (LBD), are not considered good candidates.

> • You have responded well to levodopa (i.e., your symptoms have been reduced).

> • You are now experiencing side effects of the medications, such as dyskinesia (involuntary writhing movements) or motor fluctuations (unpredictable "on" and "off" times).

> • You are 69 or younger. Patients in their 70s who have no other medical conditions and are otherwise in good health are usually considered as well.

> • You have little or no **cognitive dysfunction**. This is the most difficult and subjective criterion to assess.

Unfortunately, there are no required steps, no checklist that *must be* completed, before surgery is performed (Okun, et al., 2005). (In my opinion, this is part of the reason that some people who might not qualify under rigorous uniform standards undergo the procedure and don't get good results.)

Doctors at the University of Florida Movement Disorder Clinic have developed a questionnaire that physicians can administer in about five minutes. This tool lets doctors who are not movement disorder specialists evaluate whether to refer patients to facilities that specialize in DBS. The questionnaire is called the Florida Surgical Questionnaire for Parkinson's Disease, or FLASQ-PD, for short (Okun, Hernandez, and Foote). A copy can be found in Appendix A. It is available online.

In April 2008, Medtronic announced the U.S. premiere of its Patient Referral Advisor software (Medtronic2, 2008). This software, which is available to physicians online, uses criteria developed by a team of nine neurologists to determine the degree to which a patient is a good candidate for DBS. Your doctor might enter your specific information into this system and use the resulting recommendation as a tool for discussing the topic with you.

These tools allow patients to see and know the various criteria for surgery that are being applied to every patient who comes to that clinic for evaluation.

Right now, in many clinics, the evaluation process seems arbitrary and mysterious. I have some friends who have undergone DBS surgery, and when I've asked them how their neuropsychology testing went, they responded with puzzled looks.

Even though there are no rules or regulations, most neurosurgeons who perform DBS follow certain steps. These hold true for all types of DBS that are currently FDA-approved.

STEPS IN THE EVALUATION PROCESS

> 1. Exam by a neurologist or movement disorder specialist, specifically for the surgery. Your physician should not count your regularly scheduled ten-minute med check appointment that occurs every six months as this exam. For people with PD, this means going into the appointment off of your meds. You don't take them for at least twelve hours prior to the exam. You'll do the usual party tricks involved in a neurological exam, then take your meds, and then do the

party tricks again in an hour or so.

2. MRI (magnetic resonance imaging) of the brain
3. Exam/meeting with neurosurgeon
4. Neuropsychological examination

I know you are thinking, "The Sinemet isn't working anymore. That's why I want to have this surgery!" Your neurologist needs to know, because the goal of the surgery is to get you back to your best "on" time when your meds are working. Also, if levodopa has generally not worked for you, you may have something other than Parkinson's disease.

The brain MRI is difficult only in that you have to lie very still for a long time. Being still, even for a very short time, is hard for most of us with movement disorders. If you have a history of claustrophobia, let the radiology technician know ahead of time. Very often, the MRI personnel are allowed to give you Valium or a similar drug to help you to relax.

The neuropsych exam can be the "make-or-break" part of the evaluation process. If you show significant difficulty with cognition and memory, you will probably be excluded because DBS doesn't help those symptoms and, in some cases, appears to make them worse.

How do neuropsychologists assess your memory and cognition? With tests—lots of tests, such as asking you to:

- give the definitions of words
- repeat lists of words or numbers, backwards and forward
- answer questions about a short story you read and then
- answer them again later in the interview
- identify repeating patterns of shapes
- replicate patterns with wooden blocks in a specific amount of time (I really disliked this one)

Defining what constitutes significant problems with memory and cognition is difficult because some loss of both is considered a normal part of the aging process. Impairments in cognition and memory also are recognized as common effects of PD. The neuropsychologist can compare your results to other individuals your age to determine if there is any concern for dementia. The neuropsychological evaluation also helps determine if mood problems may interfere with your ability to safely undergo surgery. All of this information also helps to establish a baseline, in case there are changes after surgery.

You also must also be considered capable of following up after surgery for programming appointments and physician visits. This is particularly important if you live alone.

Having a history of severe depression that has not responded well to treatment can exclude you as well. I have had bouts of depression since childhood, and in my interview, the psychiatrist expressed some concern about this. I explained that historically, I have been able to recognize when I am depressed and seek treatment (such as medication or counseling) myself. I said that I believed that I could continue to do so. The psychiatrist and I agreed that seeing a therapist for a few months prior to the surgery—and continued visits after the procedure—would be an acceptable way to monitor my moods.

Chapter Six
Choosing the Team That Is Best You

More and more neurosurgeons are performing deep brain stimulation surgery every day. In my opinion, this is both a good thing and a bad thing.

It's a good thing, in that people in remote rural areas will not have to travel so far to have their surgery done; there will be a larger pool of surgeons from which to choose.

But I think it is potentially risky for patients, as the surgeon closest to them geographically may not have done many DBS surgeries and, therefore, may not be as prepared if anything out of the ordinary should happen. I also believe that surgeries already have been performed on people who never should have been considered as candidates in the first place, and having more surgeons available will make it more likely that referring physicians will err on the side of approving such patients.

I am not saying this out of malice or because I want to deprive anyone of treatment. I have known people who had noticeable cognitive problems prior to surgery, and those symptoms worsened after DBS. I have been told by recently diagnosed patients that their doctor has already told them to expect to be on medication for awhile; then, they will have DBS. This seems very irresponsible to me, since those patients haven't undergone complete evaluations.

Regardless of how many neurosurgeons are in your "neck of the woods," I believe that it is important that you feel good about having that doctor work on you, that you trust him or her. You don't necessarily have to *like* the surgeon, but you *do* need to feel comfortable that she will do her best for you.

Each person will have a different reaction to different surgeons. There is no "one size fits all" physician. So what I'm saying is, don't feel as if you have to go with the neurosurgeon to whom you are referred by your doctor.

Find out from your health insurance company or Medicare what the parameters are and then "shop around." There are some surgeons now who do bilateral DBS surgery in four stages, instead of two: 1) place the first lead in the brain; 2) implant one neurostimulator in the chest three-four weeks later and turn on the neurostimulator immediately; 3) approximately six months later, place the second lead on the other side of the brain; and 4) implant another neurostimulator or connect the second lead to the neurostimulator that has already been implanted in Step 2. Your insurance company may balk at paying for four surgeries, so be sure to check in advance.

Have a discussion with your family about the expectations that each of you has about the surgery. You should do this, even if you have decided not to look any further for a surgeon. It is important that you all know what each person expects, and that information needs to be measured against the outcomes your surgeon has said you might expect.

Here are a few questions that you might want to ask the neurosurgeon who will be sticking wires into your head. You might want to photocopy it and take a copy to appointments. (You could do the same for the programmer list that will follow.)

***

NEUROSURGEON INTERVIEW CHECKLIST

- ☐ How many times have you performed DBS surgery?

- ☐ Where were you trained to perform the surgery? Which neurosurgeon(s) trained you?

- ☐ Have you ever had a surgery with complications, such as a stroke, hemorrhage, etc.? If so, how many?

- ☐ What is the infection rate at the facility where my surgery would be performed?

- ☐ How many of your patients have developed post-surgical infections?

- ☐ Do you install the leads and the pacemaker(s) in one surgery, two, or four, and why? (There is no "right" answer to this question, but your surgeon should be able to explain to you the rationale for his or her method.)

☐ Have you had any additional training or attended any optional programming seminars? Do you read the scientific literature on DBS?

☐ If I agree to have my surgery done with your team, am I guaranteed to have you as my surgeon?

☐ When would I be likely to get on your surgery schedule?

☐ Are any of your patients willing to contact me to discuss their experience? (Because of patient confidentiality laws, your doctor cannot give you the names of his or her patients unless the patient gives express written permission. You, however, can give your contact information and permission for patients to contact you.)

☐ Do you have any information about how you and your team do the procedure at your facility?

***

An experienced neurosurgeon at a reputable facility is likely to have a considerable packet of information about what to expect from surgery, programming, and post-surgical follow-up. Even if the program is new, he should have written information about his plans and goals for care. If he doesn't, I'd be worried.

After you interview the neurosurgeons, I think it is a good idea to take some time to mull over your options. Maybe Dr. A hasn't done as many surgeries as Dr. Z, but you can get on his schedule three months sooner. Obviously, *someone* has to be the first patient on whom the surgery is performed. It's up to you whether or not you want to be that person. Or perhaps Dr. C has done a lot of DBS surgeries but you don't like his "bedside manner." Dr. Y seemed genuinely interested in you as a person and you felt that you could trust her.

Okay. You have interviewed the neurosurgeons and picked one. You're not done yet. Finding someone who can put the electrical leads in the optimal place is only half of the battle. You will need a programmer who is willing to work with you to maximize the benefits of DBS, while minimizing any side effects. That can take time, patience, and attention to your body.

As of this writing, there are no standard minimum training requirements for programmers.

Medtronic staff provides basic training only, and the growing number of neurologists, physicians, psychiatrists, and nurses who are called on to do programming makes it difficult for them to keep everyone up-to-date on the latest research and development.

Here are some questions that I would ask any potential programmer. Again, there are no "right" answers to most of these questions; it is more a matter of your comfort level.

***

CHECKLIST FOR INTERVIEWING DBS PROGRAMMERS

☐ What is your level of medical training (e.g., neurologist, nurse, physician's assistant)?

☐ When and where did you begin programming?

☐ Have you had any additional training or attended any optional programming seminars? Do you read the scientific literature on DBS?

☐ How many patients have you programmed, or how many patients are you seeing currently?

☐ Do you work under a supervising physician? If so, what is that physician's name?

☐ Everyone is different, but on average, how many times do you see a patient before you feel that his or her programming is complete?

Do you ask your patients to come back for annual checkups or wire and battery checks?

***

Best-case scenario will be that the neurosurgeon you like best will be paired with the programmer you like best. If the two don't match, I would go with the surgeon I liked. If you are unhappy with your programmer, it is much easier to switch to someone else. The DBS programmer database would be one way to locate another provider.

The Parkinson Alliance has helped to promote a voluntary Internet-based database of programmers who receive their own Web page after they register. This website was created by Sierra Farris, a DBS programmer and an advocate for patients. Patients can go to the site (www.dbsprogrammer.com) to look for programmers in their area.

Chapter Seven
"One Lump or Two?" Who Decides?

Your neurosurgeon will discuss your symptoms with you and make a recommendation about the type of system you should have.

If your symptoms are largely or exclusively on one side, you will only have one lead, with four electrodes, placed in your brain. If your symptoms affect your entire body, you will generally have two leads placed, one in the right hemisphere of your brain and one in the left.

There are two main types of neurostimulators in use today. Medtronic's Kinetra is a single unit that can be used to control each side of the brain separately. It has many advantages over the Soletra and the Itrel II, the other type of neurostimulator, which each control only one lead:

- One stimulator means fewer incisions.

- Patients have some degree of control over their settings (your programmer sets the range).

- Amplitude can be fine-tuned in small increments.

- More rate settings give programmers flexibility to use lowest beneficial amplitude.

- Patient's "**Access Therapy Controller**" can monitor battery life.

- A patient who has a cardiac pacemaker or defibrillator can still have bilateral surgery. (Stewart, Desaloms and Sanghera)

Your surgeon, however, may have reasons for using the smaller Soletra or Itrel II neurostimulators. For example, I am fairly small-boned, and my surgeon was worried that the Kinetra might be too prominent and too heavy. If there is not sufficient muscle tissue on which to attach the neurostimulator, it may slip, over time, causing the connector wire to loosen or dislodge completely. Surgery would be required to fix it. It might even become necessary to put in longer connector wires, which would mean opening up your head again. You want to avoid that, if at all possible.

Because the ANS devices are not yet approved by the Food and Drug Administration, I was unable to obtain specifics about their products. If they have received FDA approval by the time you read this, I would consider asking if their devices come in different sizes.

Chapter Eight
DBS: The Paperwork

When investigating your eligibility with your doctor, it's a good idea to make sure that your insurance, if you have it, will cover DBS. Most insurance companies do, but they generally want you to be pre-approved.

There may also be other stipulations, such as sharing a room, unless there are only private rooms available, or limiting the number of days you can be hospitalized.

This surgery is expensive! I've heard a range from $60,000 to $150,000. Most procedures are somewhere in between. This figure does not include the costs related to the evaluation, the pre-op physical, or the programming. A number of factors affect the price of the surgery:

- The level of expertise of the surgeon

- The size of the surgical team

- The length of the surgery, which depends on your brain's anatomy, the surgeon's precision in placing the lead(s), and possible complications

- Post-operative pain issues (If you are in a lot of pain, your doctor will provide stronger pain medication, but often, it has to be administered through an IV, which means you have to stay in the hospital.)

- Other arcane and seemingly arbitrary fees that the hospital charges

I speak from experience when I say it is a good idea to write down or get written copies of any steps that you must take before the surgery and your hospital stays. Also make note of the date you called and the name of the person with whom you spoke.

Medicare does cover DBS, but each state may have its own rules about how to qualify.

The insurance issue can be addressed before or during the evaluation process, but you will be required to tell your doctor who is going to pay for the surgery before he or she will do it.

If cost is an issue, look for opportunities to participate in clinical trials. There are currently a number of research studies seeking patients to undergo DBS surgery in order to evaluate techniques, products, or efficacy. Generally, when you participate in a clinical trial, your surgical costs are covered. Other expenses may be covered as well.

Make sure your insurance will cover the programming after surgery. Some insurance companies are limiting how much time the programmer can spend in trying to get the best settings. Twenty five hours the first year would not be unusual.

Warning! Read the Fine Print

My husband's health plan, which supplies my coverage, changed on January 1, 2007. We learned the hard way that it is not enough to see a doctor in the system. For example, we have to call Company E to verify that the clinician we want to see is approved for coverage at that location. If my doctor orders any tests, I need to ask whether or not those services are contracted out. This includes x-rays, MRIs, CT scans—all of the diagnostic imaging. If the service is provided by someone else, I have to call again. When the provider is in-network, Company E pays 80 percent, and we pay 20 percent. For out-of-network services, they pay 60 percent—after we have exceeded a $3000 family deductible—and we pay 40 percent.

I am writing about this partly because I need to do some spleen-venting. With DBS, there are so many tests that need to be done before and during the procedure. You need to find out exactly what your insurance company means if it indicates that the surgery is "covered." Otherwise, you could find yourself facing some hefty bills that were unexpected.

DBS AND INCOME TAXES: SAVE ALL RECEIPTS!

If you itemize your tax return *and* your medical expenses for the tax year exceed 7.5 percent of your adjusted gross income, you can deduct a portion of those medical expenses from your federal income tax.[1]

Because I chose to have my surgery done in Cleveland, which is a twelve-hour drive or a two-hour plane ride from Minneapolis, my medical travel expenses were considerable. I couldn't deduct meals or entertainment, but I could claim transportation (including mileage and parking) and lodging.

Even if you don't travel far for your surgery, it makes sense to save your receipts from parking or cab fare for doctor appointments. They add up quickly, especially over the course of a year. An easy way to figure mileage without leaving the house is to use Mapquest.com or some other Internet mapping program. Enter your address and your doctor's address. Then multiply that number by two to get the mileage for one round-trip. Multiply that number times the number of doctor visits on your calendar for the tax year.

1   *Medical and Dental Expenses*. Internal Revenue Service Publication, 2007, 502.

Chapter Nine
"Anticipa-a-tion":
The Countdown to Surgery

The amount of time between evaluation and surgery can vary widely. It depends on many factors, including the surgeon's schedule. If the neurosurgeon you choose is in demand, you may have to wait several weeks. A surgeon who is newer to the surgery will probably have openings more quickly. Your health is also a factor. If you have a cold, or the flu, or a flare-up of a chronic condition, you may have to wait up to thirty days after full recovery before having DBS.

Some prescription medications, such as blood thinners (e.g., Coumadin, aspirin), must be stopped at least ten days prior to surgery—this reduces the risk of a brain hemorrhage or stroke.

As you will see by my blog entry, I had to wait awhile for my surgery. In fact, it was around five months from the date of my initial consultation with my primary movement disorder specialist to the date of my lead implantation surgery. Most neurosurgeons can schedule the procedure more quickly.

One Week from Today!
Tuesday, January 10, 2006

I have never been good at waiting, so this time until the surgery actually happens is really a challenge.

Over the past few days, I have spoken at length with three other people who have been through DBS surgery. These conversations have reinforced my beliefs that I am doing the right thing and at the right place. The trick now is balancing realistic expectations with wild hopes and worries about complications.

Last night, we talked some more with the boys about what will happen during the operations and about how it will take a while (several months or more) to know the full effects of them.

Alex said something like, "Well, that's not worth it then!" but we reminded him that we do know that things aren't working the way they are. I don't think Bennett really grasped what we were saying, and we'll just have to see how he does.

I firmly believe that the decision of whether or not to have deep brain stimulation surgery should be the patient's, and the patient's alone. Of course, it only makes sense to take your care partner's feelings and those of other family and friends into account. But in the end, the Parkie is going to have to deal with all of the challenges.

I am so glad that my husband, Paul, let me make the decision on my own. I didn't feel any pressure to do it "for" him, and that helped a lot. The decision to see if you are a candidate for brain surgery is stressful enough without [added] pressure from loved ones or even your employer.

From First Symptoms to Surgery: My Timeline
Saturday, December 24, 2005

In case you are thinking "Wow, this is all happening really fast!" or "What's taking so long?" here is a timeline to let you know where things stand.

January 1997 - I noticed my first symptoms—stiffening/lack of control in my left pinkie and ring fingers—when I returned to work after Bennett's birth. (In hindsight, there were signs long before; I just didn't recognize them.)

July 1998 - About eighteen months and three neurologists later, I was diagnosed with "hemi-parkinsonism" (parkinsonian symptoms on one side of the body). I started Sinemet then, and have been on it ever since.

Fall 2001 - The first of many members of my support group to undergo DBS has her surgery. Her extreme tremors are nearly gone, and she can write and drive again, but I can't get past the fact that her surgeon didn't recall the operation in which he implanted her pacemakers!

30

June 2004 - I left my position as co-director of the Food & Health Program at the Institute for Agriculture and Trade Policy to go on long-term disability. My neurologist had been advising this for more than two years.

August 2005 - A phone call from ABC-TV, combined with some freezing episodes, *really* bad dyskinesia, and fluctuations in on/ off time, led to my decision to consider DBS.

Paul and I saw my neurologist, who, after making me perform the standard neurological "party tricks," pronounced me an "excellent candidate" for surgery. He wrote up the paperwork and insurance referrals, and we were on our way.

I had a brain MRI done at the University of Minnesota. I was afraid that the radiology techs would have to give me Valium or else re-do the scans because of my dyskinesia, but apparently all of those Velcro straps on the exam table and the "vise" for my head did the trick!

Early September 2005 - It wasn't a matter of having specific misgivings about the U of M's DBS program; I just didn't feel an innate sense of trust and confidence. After thinking about this for more than three years, I felt that I needed to have complete and total faith in my surgeon.

I talked with several people, and Dr. Ali Rezai at Cleveland Clinic was mentioned several times. I contacted the Parkinson Alliance, which hosts the DBS-STN.org website, to see if they had any statistics on rates of complications and infections at various hospitals around the country. They don't, but CEO Carol Walton encouraged me to do thorough research to make sure I was comfortable with my choice. She also gave me some names of patients who'd undergone DBS, in case I wanted to chat with them about their experiences.

I talked with several people who had been patients of Dr. Rezai and were very happy with their results. I contacted the Center for Neurological Restoration at the Cleveland Clinic and liked what I heard, so I made an appointment.

September 29, 2005 - I was able to get two of the three

necessary appointments scheduled for the end of September. (I would've had to wait until the end of December to find a date for which all three could be scheduled. That seemed like too long, so I agreed to a separate trip.)

Paul and I met with Dr. Monique Giroux that morning. I had to go in without meds so that she could see how well/poorly I functioned without Sinemet. Then, after taking my meds, I got to do the party tricks again. She asked, "What took you so long?" to consider surgery.

That day, we also met with the neurosurgeon, Dr. Ali Rezai, and with Sierra Farris, one of the programmers. We were very impressed with everyone, especially Dr. Rezai, who has done more than five hundred DBS surgeries himself! He also said I was an "excellent candidate." Last stop, neuropsych!

October 20, 2005 - Four hours of neuropsych and cognitive testing! Yuck! (Actually, some of the word games were fun, but reciting lists of numbers backwards and copying shapes with blocks got old pretty fast). I think that these tests showed that I still have most of my marbles and so should be eligible for the surgery. I also met with Dr. Cynthia Kubu, who did a psych evaluation. We talked about my history of depression, which has responded to medication and which I have always recognized and sought treatment. We also discussed that what I'm feeling now is not like past episodes of depression, in which I haven't felt motivated to do anything. Now I *want* to do things, but my body won't let me. Big difference!

I had to go back on medication for my Crohn's disease (digestive disorder), but it's not steroids this time, so I don't *think* it will present a problem for surgery.

November 2005 - Lots of waiting! When are they going to call me with a surgery date? Also got a letter from Dr. Kubu stating that in light of my past depression, I should go back to seeing my psychologist before the surgery and continue afterward. This way, I can be monitored for any psych/cognitive/behavior changes.

December 2005 - Finally, a surgery date! First, it was January 31. Later, it was moved up to Tuesday, January 17. Now, we were finally able to start making plans for child care, etc.

January 5, 2006 - I have to go to Cleveland for my pre-op physical. I had hoped to do most of it here, and have the rest done there on the day before surgery. However, because of the Crohn's disease, I will go meet with the gastroenterologist to make sure I'm okay on that front. That way, if there is a concern, I have a couple of weeks to make it go away.

January 16, 2006 - Check in to the hospital. Say good-bye to my hair!

January 17, 2006 - Lead placement surgery. I'll be awake for this, to help the docs make sure they're working on the right spots in my brain. I'll be in a stereotactic frame, or "halo," so that I'm not wiggling all over the place.
No airplane flights for seven days because the combination of brain swelling and atmospheric pressure changes could be catastrophic! So we will stay in Cleveland to sample its tourist attractions. Rock and Roll Hall of Fame, here we come!

January 23, 2006 - Pacemakers are put in place. This surgery is performed under general anesthetic but once it's done, I can leave the hospital. If it's late in the day, I'll probably stay in until the next day, but then it will be time to go home!

February 17, 2006 (approx.) - Back to Cleveland to have the system turned on and receive the initial programming. (Each surgery center may have a different approach to the number of surgeries and the timing of turning on the device. Although I am anxious to experience the results, I like the idea of giving my body some time to get used to the new hardware!)

February 18-21, 2006 - Parkinson's Action Network policy forum and state/congressional coordinators meeting in Washington DC. I plan to be there!

February 22-26, 2006 - The World Parkinson's Congress is also being held in DC, right after the PAN forum. I am very excited (and nervous) about my two poster sessions on advocacy and my poem and sculpture that will appear in the "Creativity and PD" exhibit.

Mid-March through mid-July 2006 - I will be going back to Cleveland approximately once a month for programming until it is optimized. That will probably be about six months.

Chapter Ten
Preparing Yourself Psychologically

Depending on your health, your surgeon's schedule, weather, and other things beyond your control, you will most likely have to wait a couple of weeks—or even several months. You can use that time wisely by preparing yourself emotionally for what is to come.

Of course you are nervous! This is brain surgery, after all. But you will have some control over the outcome if you go in with a positive attitude. I'm not saying you will be able to come out of the surgery with everything the way it was before you had any PD symptoms, but you can visualize yourself walking unaided, chopping vegetables without a box of Band-Aids next to you, figure skating—doing something that you used to be able to do while you were "on" reliably.

I am one of those people who cannot relax by herself; I need someone to tell me what to do. I found a book, *Prepare for Surgery, Heal Faster* by Peggy Huddleston, very helpful as I tried to relax and visualize a good surgical outcome. The book came with guided meditations on CD. The package offered tips for staying positive and expecting a good outcome. For example, following her instructions, I wrote a note stating that the surgery would go well, my pain would be manageable, and my voice would be clear and strong. I taped the note to my gown so that my doctors would see it during surgery. (I asked them to read it aloud while I was sedated, but I don't think it happened. They seemed to find the idea a bit silly.)

I Made It through Christmas!
Monday, December 26, 2005

I am very happy to report that I made it through Christmas Eve and Christmas Day without any major medication meltdowns!

Last week, I tended to stiffen up in the late afternoons, and the Sinemet didn't help a lot. This made doing things like attending my boss' birthday party quite a challenge. Everyone told me I *looked* great (dyskinesia is a very effective weight-loss "program"), and they assumed that since I wasn't wiggling all over, that I was doing well, when really, I was very uncomfortable from the stiffness.

I have been very glad that so far on this trip down to Jackson (we drove down from the Twin Cities yesterday), my dyskinesia has been reasonably under control. When we were here over Thanksgiving, I think that I wiggled off about five pounds in two days, despite eating everything in sight.

Three Weeks from Today
Tuesday, December 27, 2005

Exactly three weeks from right now, I plan to be resting comfortably in the hospital at Cleveland Clinic after a successful surgery to put the leads in place for the DBS unit! I have been listening to the relaxation CD that is a companion to the *Prepare for Surgery, Heal Faster* book. Hopefully, that will help me to keep from worrying myself into a meltdown.

I scored big at ARC Value Village today! I needed to get some pants that fit (I've wiggled off a couple more pounds) and tops without buttons (too much fine-motor control required). Thank goodness for thrift stores and garage sales because in the nine years I've had PD and Crohn's, I've experienced a sixty-pound range of weight gain/loss! My neurologist warned me that most DBS patients gain ten to fifteen pounds in the first six to twelve months after the surgery, largely due to decreased dyskinesia, so I'll be holding on to the clothes that are currently too big. Because I've always been a "fashion don't" (you may remember how *Glamour* magazine used to have a section with photos of women wearing the "right" clothes—the "fashion do's"—and those wearing the "wrong" clothes—the "fashion don'ts"), I'm not too worried about being out of style.

~ * ~

I resolve to be more positive in '06
Sunday, January 1, 2006

I continue to learn how important attitude is with this disease. For so long, I was extremely negative ("The glass is not only half-empty; it's cracked, too"), and I know that I still have that tendency. Some of that is probably genetic, since one of Great-Grandma Willett's famous sayings was "If it's not one thing, it's two!"

However, I am trying very hard to focus on what I have and what I can do, rather than what I lack and can no longer do. I have an amazing husband and two wonderful sons, along with scores of loving and generous family members and friends who have been showering me with love, prayers, gifts, and more.

I am blessed to be eligible for the DBS surgery. Not all Parkies are good candidates for the procedure. I have health insurance that is supposed to cover the operation, and top-notch doctors and nurses to take care of me.

I can still type (although writing this takes an embarrassingly long time), and I have the tools to do it. I just need to remember the song at the end of the Monty Python movie The Meaning of Life—"Always Look on the Bright Side of Life." (I must remember to add that to my list of songs that I want playing during my surgery!)

This entry makes me think about one of the things I enjoyed so much about the neurosurgery team at Cleveland Clinic: the staff allow patients to supply their own music (if they choose to do so; it isn't necessary) to be played in the operating room during the times when they are awake and being stitched up (e.g., between "sides" of the brain). This made me feel so much more comfortable and comforted. I think it was the anesthesiologist who said he liked the mix I had created for the occasion.

Check to see if your surgeon has a similar policy about music, and make tapes or CDs. You also could collect soothing music or books on tape to be played while you are convalescing.

If possible, "hold court." Ask friends and relatives to come to see you. The purpose of this is twofold: If, heaven forbid, something goes wrong during the surgery, everyone will be glad that they saw you. And on a much more positive note, you will want them to be able to see the likely very stark contrast in your symptoms that will be apparent within weeks or months of the surgery! Be sure to avoid people with colds, strep throat, or the flu. You don't want illness to delay your surgery.

Chapter Eleven
Logistical Tasks to Be Completed before Surgery

The previous chapter listed things to do to pass the time. Here are some tasks that are prudent, if not legally required.

1) **Make a will,** or review your current one and update it, if necessary. There are a number of law offices that are relatively inexpensive (about $100–$150 here in Minneapolis in 2008). If you can't afford to see a lawyer or prefer to do it yourself, there are also boilerplate legal forms that you can buy online. The same is true for advance medical directive forms. Get the correct documents for your state, and fill in the blanks with your information. Get it notarized, or have it properly witnessed. Put a copy of the will into a safe deposit box.

2) **Make an advance medical directive** (a legal document that indicates what you do and do not want done in case there are complications). It's good to have one even if you are not facing brain surgery. Think about whether or not you want to have a DNR ("do not resuscitate" order. Get the document prepared (it has to be witnessed and notarized). Have copies made to give to your care team and to put in your medical record and in your safe deposit box.

Doing these things may seem morbid and depressing, but they need to be done, and sometimes it takes a major life event, such as brain surgery, to give us the impetus to actually make a will or sign up to donate our brains for research when we die. The risk of dying because of DBS surgery, however, is very, very low.

3) **Have a dental checkup** and get any necessary dental work done prior to surgery. Women should have a mammogram. (It is still possible to have it done afterward, but take it from me—it will be much easier and more

comfortable if you do it prior to surgery.)

4) Make a care plan. Write it out and make copies for everyone involved. The plan should address all of the following questions that apply to you. (Note: I am putting this into a checklist so that you can make copies for everyone involved.)

- Who will be with you at the hospital?
- Who will make sure that you get your medications on time and in the correct amounts?
- Who will house-sit for you?
- Who will take care of your kids (depending on your age and theirs) or your pets?
- Who will drive you home from the hospital?
- Who will help you with household chores (you are not supposed to raise your arms above your head for several days or to lift anything more than a pound or two for a couple of weeks)?

All of these questions represent needs that must be met to ensure a safe surgical experience and period of recuperation.

Neurologists may try to discourage someone from having the surgery if he or she lives alone and has no family, friends, or neighbors who can help with these tasks. If you fall into that category, try contacting United Way's First Call for Help, usually listed in the front few pages of your telephone book. If you are or have been involved in a church, there is most likely a committee dedicated to serving people in your situation.

Figure 2

DBS CARE PLAN

Hospital Companions

Lead placement surgery (Ask your surgeon to ESTIMATE length of surgery)

Date	Time slot	Name	Phone number(s)
25-Jun	6:00-7:00 a.m.	John Smith	612-555-1111 (home); 651-555-1111 (cell)

After surgery

Medication Monitor While I Am Hospitalized

Make sure that Parkinson medication & other prescriptions are given according to patient's drug schedule

Housesitter(s)

Babysitters & Petsitter(s)

Post-Op Drivers

Figure 3

DBS CARE PLAN
Page 2

Meals

For family while I'm in the hospital

Date	Meal time	Name	Phone number(s)	Food brought	Return dishes?
25-Jun	Dinner	John Smith	612-555-1111 (home)	Tuna casserole & salad	No

For when I return home or for freezer during recuperation

Date	Meal time	Name	Phone number(s)	Food brought	Return dishes?

Things We Need Help with Before, During and After Surgery
Saturday, December 24, 2005

Needs

This is a very difficult list for me to make, because I hate asking for help, but we need some assistance with the following:

- Driving Paul's carpool shifts from school on Tuesday, Thursday, and Friday afternoons while we're out of town
- Taking Bennett to tae kwon do from 5:30 to 6:30, two nights/week
- Shoveling/blowing snow, if necessary
- Meals (frozen or instant) while we're out of town and when we first get back
- Assistance with laundry and cleaning while we're in Cleveland
- Play dates/outings for Alex and Bennett

So Many People Who Want to Help

I am still feeling rather awestruck and overwhelmed by the number of people who want to help us get through this latest PD challenge! I think I am going to be receiving more prayers, energy, light, and good thoughts than any patient they've ever had at Cleveland Clinic!

Last night, I was on the receiving end of a healing touch/energy work session with two of my aunts and two of my cousins. I think they generated enough energy to light the entire Twin Cities! It was truly an amazing phenomenon. During the session, I kept hearing soothing voices (not those of my family) telling me, "We're always with you. Everything is going to be okay. Nothing bad is going to happen; you've got a lot of work to do here. You just don't have to be sick to do it." I felt as if a huge weight had been lifted off of me.

Some of you may think that this is proof that I've finally gone off the deep end, and that certainly is a possibility. But I feel like it was a real breakthrough for me, and I interpret the experience as further confirmation that I'm doing the right thing.

Asking for help around the house during and after my surgeries was one of the hardest things I've had to do since developing PD. What finally helped me to "let it go" was the realization (which was pointed out by my therapist) that it was the only way for most of the people who love me to express that love.

Some of the favors we needed from family and friends were significant. For example, we needed someone to stay with our kids so that Paul could be with me. We ended up asking Paul's sister, Annie. It was a big deal for her to come from Portland, Oregon, for ten days, but we knew that the kids would be much more relaxed than if we hired a babysitter. Luckily, Annie and her husband, Scott, who make Raptor Ridge wines, have clients in Minnesota, so Annie was able to do some work while she was here.

Sometimes, people come up with ways to help that you might not have identified yourself. Kari Huseth, a high school friend whom I hadn't seen in years, called out of the blue to offer her services as a certified nursing assistant. She offered to fly to Cleveland and drive back with us. This turned out to be a godsend! She knew that I needed to keep my pain under control and woke me up during the night to take pain meds; helped me to get dressed; and even convinced Paul to stop for the night on our way back home because she saw that I was in so much pain.

Of course, not everyone could commit to these major favors. They couldn't come along to Cleveland to hold my hand; they couldn't take the Parkinson's or the pain away, but by God, they could make a hot dish for Annie and the boys! Those meals were such a lifesaver for Annie, as well as for Paul and me when we returned home. And I am eternally grateful to my friend Kathy Hiltsley, who agreed to coordinate the list of meals and volunteers.

Chapter Twelve
Talking to Kids about Deep Brain Stimulation

As I've said, when my husband and I talked with our kids about the possibility of my undergoing DBS, they had two very different responses. Alex said, "Go for it!" while Bennett said, "What if something goes wrong?" I am no child psychologist, but I think that those responses are very common.

Older children, especially those who have watched you suffer for a long time, may share your desperation to try almost anything for some relief. It is only natural to ask yourself about the possibility of surgical complications, but I think it is important to be honest with your child or children, without going into a lot of specifics.

Our kids almost always have a better idea of what is going on with the family than we parents are willing to acknowledge. We encouraged our sons to ask as many questions as they wanted. I learned that I needed to explain the process using everyday language, stop frequently for questions, and most of all, listen carefully. If they asked a question such as, "What will they do at the hospital?" and I launched into a very detailed account of the procedure, I might only get as far as "The doctor will put me to sleep and then ..." before they had moved on to "Can I play soccer tonight?" When kids change the subject, it usually means that their question has been answered to their satisfaction, and they do not want additional information.

Personally, I would not go into extreme detail about the procedures unless I was talking to a college student, and then only if asked. I found that my older son, Alex, who was 14 when I had surgery, had questions like "Are there wires sticking out of your head?" when I talked to him from the hospital. He didn't want to hear about the process of putting on the stereotactic frame ("halo").

Just as young children have trouble understanding why you still have Parkinson's disease after a long time has passed—after all, they get colds or the flu and recover quickly—they also may expect you to return home completely recovered. After all, that's what happens on TV shows: everything is all fixed by the end of the episode.

My children, especially my younger son, Bennett, had difficulty understanding why I needed to continue to make programming trips to Cleveland. The surgery was over. Hadn't it fixed everything? Not quite.

It is difficult to find an analogy that could help to explain the situation to kids, but they might relate to this one. Say they have very crooked teeth and have been told they need braces. First, they have to have some teeth pulled. Next, they get braces put on their remaining teeth. But if the metal bands are not tightened regularly, the teeth will not get moved into the proper places. And even then, after the braces come off, teeth may move out of place again. It's not an ideal analogy, but is probably one that older children could understand, as you are trying to make the point that DBS is a process, and not a perfect one at that.

We also chose to enlist the help of a psychologist who specialized in play therapy to help Bennett in dealing with his feelings about my PD and the surgery. Don't be afraid to ask for help! Parenting is tough enough under normal circumstances. There is no shame in acknowledging that chronic illness adds a high degree of difficulty to the job.

Chapter Thirteen
Telling Family and Friends

Telling your family and friends is a very personal choice, so I am only making recommendations. I don't believe there is a template for dealing with issues like this.

Prior to the surgery, I personally told my parents, in-laws, two brothers, four aunts with whom I am close, three college friends, some work colleagues, members of our support group, and several Parkie friends.

Because my surgery was going to occur just after the New Year, and I hadn't had time to send Christmas cards, I sent a holiday letter and included a paragraph about the surgery.

Immediately after the surgery, it will be obvious that you've "had some work done." You will have either a shaved head or "racing stripes" shorn through your hair. Depending on how much you are out and about and how comfortable you are discussing your surgery with strangers, it is completely your decision whether to explain DBS to the grocery clerk, for example; you are under no obligation to do so.

In my book *The First Year: Parkinson's Disease*, I wrote of the question that most Parkies have come to dread: "How are you?" I wrote that it is up to us to decide whether we respond with a report on our PD, or on our mood, or life in general.

If you are asked, "No, really, how *are* you?" it's a safe bet this person wants the PD update, and you can either tell him or her, or politely say something like, "It's been a long day. I'd rather not talk about Parkinson's right now."

Everybody who had seen me prior to DBS has noticed a change—I'm no longer wiggling like a human Slinky—so when they say, "You look great!" I am thrilled to tell them about the surgery.

December 17—Thirty Days to Surgery
Saturday, December 17, 2005

Wow, it's hard to believe that my deep brain stimulation surgery (DBS) is just thirty days away. Words that describe how I feel: excited, terrified, hopeful, anxious, blessed, squeamish, lucky. Those are some that immediately spring to mind.

Although January in the Midwest may not seem like the best time to undergo brain surgery (is there ever a good time for brain surgery?), I can take heart in the fact that I won't be the only one wearing a hat. There are many stylish and silly hats available. And I can always indulge my hairdresser's suggestion that I experiment with wigs!

The fact that this time immediately preceding the surgery is also the December holiday season gives me license to contact old friends, rarely seen relatives, and work colleagues about my impending life change in a slightly less artificial way. They're expecting a holiday card or note from me anyway. Granted, they're not expecting one that says "Happy holidays! What's new with you? I'm having brain surgery in a month!" but hey, it's better than dealing with all of the complaints of "Why didn't you tell me?" after the fact, and it gives me a reason to let them know I'm thinking about them and value our relationship—something I should do anyway, but I guess I've needed a little nudge from the universe. I'm going to hug my husband and kids now ... More later.

~*~

PREPARATIONS FOR THE "BIG DAY"
Off to Cleveland tomorrow for Thurs. pre-op physical
Tuesday, January 3, 2006

Tomorrow (Wed. 1/4), I fly to Cleveland (via Chicago because Northwest continues to gouge people with their hideously overpriced non-stop flights). I will spend all day Thursday at seven various and sundry appointments, including EKG, lab, gastroenterology and more! My last appointment is at 3:30, and I really hope that it is on time. My flight out is at 7:50, so I should be okay, but I would hate to have to stay over another night.

Today I had lunch with my friend Kathy to go over the list of ways that folks can help us. That was hard! She is willing to be one of the "point people" here at home to monitor the process, but there are so many unknowns. The largest one is how Bennett, who is 9, will deal with both of us being away from home (he's used to my being gone but not Paul). I just need to keep reminding myself that they are both wonderful, resilient kids who know how much we love them.

~*~

Back from Cleveland—Everything is a "go"
Thursday, January 5, 2006

I just have to stay healthy between now and then. No colds or flu. This means that before bed tonight, I need to steam out my sinuses to keep them in shape.

What a long day! I definitely should have had someone with me. Lots of details to keep track of, but for now I need to get ready for bed!

~*~

Pre-op Physical Report
Friday, January 6, 2006

I started off my day at the clinic with an EKG. The technician kept saying, "Hold still. Just relax!" I had two thoughts, which I managed to keep to myself:
1) "If I could hold still whenever I wanted to, I wouldn't be here in Cleveland!"
2) "Lady, if you think I'm squirmy now, you ain't seen nothin' yet!"

At that time, I really was very still. Next, a nurse reviewed my meds and medical history. Then I chatted briefly with an internist who said if the sinus headache I was experiencing became an infection and required antibiotics, that the surgery would have to be delayed a month. So we're not going to let an infection develop!

Of course, just to keep things interesting, my dyskinesia kicked in big time, just in time for the lab work. Somehow the phlebotomist drawing the blood got the four tubes she needed.

48

Then she handed me a Styrofoam cup and a plastic vial with my medical info on it and pointed me to the ladies room. She asked if I wanted her to do the transfer from the cup to the vial but I stubbornly said no. It was touch-and-go, but I did manage to pour the urine into the vial and screw on the lid without incident.

... Lunch was a fiasco. The layout of the cafeteria is not at all conducive to people with wheelchairs, walkers, or any motor impairment. (I brought my four-wheeled walker, Lilybelle, with me. She came in very handy!) Once I got some food in a foam clamshell, I looked for a place to sit. The aisles between the tables are virtually nonexistent, let alone wide enough for a walker. However, just as I was about to give up and leave the cafeteria, a seat along the periphery of the tables opened up. The mac-and-cheese that I'd selected (comfort food) was dreadful, which was just as well. I need to watch my dairy intake to keep my sinuses clear.

Lilybelle and I schlepped my luggage along to the MRI dept. I showed up ninety minutes early, hoping to get an earlier appointment but as it was, I got done with only enough time to get to my last appointment at 3:30, which was with Ellen, who coordinates the surgery schedule and lots of other things.

The MRI was loud but very quick, and Ellen said it looked good, so I don't have to do another one on the day of surgery. Hurray! Lab work also came back fine.

Coming up next ... preparing for surgery! Ellen tells me the plan.

AN IMPORTANT REMINDER FOR PEOPLE WITH PD AND THEIR FAMILIES

Regular hospital personnel are not accustomed to dealing with Parkies. It was very difficult for me to remember that. Just as so many other members of the public don't understand why we can't sit still, the average lab tech or nurse can't figure out why we can't move our bodies across a gurney or hold still for an EKG.

This brings up two more important points. First, make multiple copies of your medication schedule so that there is one in your chart, one for your surgeon, and extras with your care partner. And second, make sure that your care partner or whoever is going to be with you at the hospital has extra doses of your medications! They may come in handy. There will be times when you will need your Sinemet and the nurse will say, "I'm sorry. That wasn't ordered. Let me contact your doctor to ask him to order it for you."

Chapter Fourteen
The Big Day

If I've learned anything at all about DBS since I've had the surgery, it's that DBS is a process, not an event.

There are at least three milestones within the DBS process. The first is the lead placement, or the brain surgery part, also known as "the part where you have to be awake."

The second milestone is the pacemaker installation, which is done under general anesthetic. Some surgeons combine one lead placement with one pacemaker installation in one long operation.

Milestone number three is turning on the system. This is when you begin to get some sense of how this thing can help you. Some surgeons will place the leads, wait three to five weeks to do the neurostimulators, and then immediately turn on the stimulation. Others implant the neurostimulators a week after leads are implanted but wait three to four weeks to turn on the system. Still other surgeons do four surgeries to complete bilateral stimulation.

As I've said before, any neurosurgeon with whom you speak should be able to tell you how he handles these three milestones—and why he does it that way.

TENTATIVE SCHEDULE OF EVENTS FOR JANUARY 16–18
Saturday, January 7, 2006
When I met with Ellen this past Thursday for my physical, she went over the schedule for the surgery. It will go something like this:

> **Monday, 1/16**—check into the hospital in the afternoon. Paul and my mom will be staying at a downtown hotel that has free shuttle service to the clinic.

Tuesday, 1/17—Mom and Paul will have to be there bright and early—5:30—to see me before I go off to get my head shaved and the stereotactic frame ("halo") put on. Then I'll have a CT scan. I'll get to see Mom and Paul briefly before going in to have my skull "prepared" for the operation. (I get to be lightly sedated for that part). The surgical team will have a meeting to go over the MRI from Thursday and the CT scan to decide where they want to implant the leads.

Once they've decided where they want to go, they'll use a probe to get to the right spots. Here's where the "party tricks" come in—the ones that make me feel like a circus animal. "Wiggle your toes for me. Tap your thumb and forefinger together as quickly as you can. Count backwards from 100 by sevens." I know that they need to do this to make sure they are affecting the parts of the brain that we want to affect and not impair the ones that are working.

I get to have music playing while all of this is happening so that will be a welcome distraction, I think. I have plenty of ideas of what I'd like to have playing, but I'm also open to suggestions.

Once they've found the sweet spot on Side A, they will insert the actual lead with its four electrodes. Then they close up Side A. (I get to take another nap). Then they do the same thing on Side B. The other ends of the leads will stop behind my ears.

The average time that it takes to go from the holes in the skull to closing up is five to eight hours. After the surgery, I'll go to the recovery room and spend the night in ICU. I'll get to see Mom and Paul for a few minutes.

The next day, I should be transferred to a regular room, and, hopefully, get "sprung" on Thursday.

Chapter Fifteen
Potential Risks and Complications of DBS Surgery

Noted environmentalist and former presidential candidate Barry Commoner once said, "There is no such thing as a free lunch." One cannot expect to undergo brain surgery without the potential for things to go wrong. With DBS, as with any brain surgery, bleeding in the brain, or a "stroke," and infection are the two biggest risks.

The occurrence of an intracranial hemorrhage, also known as bleeding within the brain, can run quite a gamut. Often, there is very little bleeding—just pinpoints of blood. These appear to have no lasting effects. Sometimes, though, surgeons may encounter a blood vessel where they did not expect to find one, or there is a sudden drastic increase in blood pressure. The pre-op physical and the brain MRI and CT scans that are done before and during the surgery give the neurosurgeon and his or her team some idea of how the body is responding to the procedure.

Strokes can be very debilitating—even more so than Parkinson's—and may be fatal. In facilities that perform a lot of DBS surgeries, however, the risk of having a stroke as a result of the operation "is usually less than 2 percent" (Kaiser Permanente). Someone suffering a mild stroke during DBS surgery might make a full recovery but still have PD. I understand that most neurosurgeons will not perform DBS surgery on someone who has a history of uncontrolled high blood pressure or stroke.

Infections are becoming all too common with any type of surgery. The risk is multiplied whenever a foreign object is implanted in the body. With DBS, that means there are several opportunities: the electrical leads, the extension wires, and the neurostimulator(s).

Nosocomial (hospital-acquired) **infections** are on the rise around the country, as are the number of infections that are resistant to many traditional antibiotics (Diekema, 2004). During your evaluation appointment, you can ask the neurosurgeon about the infection rate at his or her facility. While it is unlikely that physicians would have up-to-the-minute statistics for their hospital at their fingertips, all clinicians should be aware of infection control procedures; if they don't, I would take that as a bad sign. The DBS team should know how many infections occurred over the past year, due to the frequent follow-up required for an infection. They generally will remember the patients who had complications because of the extra care they require and because of their frequent trips back to see the DBS team. A 2005 fact sheet by Kaiser Permanente Northern California stated that the risk of serious infection (at that time) was at least 5 percent.

Of course, the responsibility for preventing infection does not lie solely with hospital staff. You should receive instructions on wound care upon your discharge. Be sure that you follow the instructions, and don't be afraid to call if you even *suspect* that you might have an infection.

Figure 4.

Signs of Infection

- Severe and persistent headache

- Redness or increased swelling around incision

- Fever of 101°F or above

- Bleeding from incision(s)

- Vision loss or changes in vision

- Chills

Call your neurosurgeon or their designated contact immediately if you experience any of these symptoms.

http://www.webmd.com/parkinsons-disease/deep-brain-stimulation?page=4, 2005-2008. Accessed June 11, 2008

One Family's Experience with Infection

My father has had other minor surgeries (hernia, for example) for which the docs had him shower for a couple days prior to surgery with surgical antibacterial soap. They did not, however, have him do that prior to DBS surgery—and so, it slipped his mind and he didn't. We do not know if that would have prevented his subsequent staph infection, but for the next surgery, his infection-control docs said it would a good idea to shower with antibacterial soap, and gave us a few other ideas for preparing for surgery.

One was to try to improve his sleep (he rarely gets more than three hours of sleep a night) so that he would be stronger and better able to fight off unwanted bacteria. We are working on other ways to beef up his immune system.

The docs have also recommended an antibacterial ointment to rub into my dad's nose prior to surgery—again, to reduce a possible infection.

Although this [DBS] is considered a fairly low-risk surgery—considering it is brain surgery, after all—patients should really consider the "what if": What if there are complications? What will we do?

Medicare would not pay for the six weeks of home-infusion antibiotics that my dad required after surgery. Luckily, his secondary insurance paid 100 percent. But if that had not been the case, he may have had to remain in the hospital for six weeks (it is our understanding that Medicare would have paid for that), or he would have had to go into a clinic four times a day, every day, for six weeks. Not very good options.

So while we wouldn't say that patients should get overly worked up about complications, there should be some serious discussions about "what if" so that they have a plan in place, if needed. That sense of control would have helped us, but we had very optimistically ruled out any real chance of complications—and were really punched in the gut when complications arose. We were just lucky that his [her father's] insurance covered everything, so that we weren't dealt an additional nightmare on the financial side of things.

Air can enter the area between the brain and the skull during surgery when dime-sized holes are made in the skull for lead placement. This trapped air can cause confusion for up to a couple of weeks after surgery. In extreme cases, it can delay post-operative waking. It is especially important that you don't fly for at least seven days after the lead placement surgery. The change in air pressure during air travel would cause undue pressure on the brain that could cause a stroke or even death.

I recently heard a very disconcerting report from a clinician at a facility that sees a lot of DBS patients. A family had made an appointment there, after a family member had DBS surgery done at a newer institution. The family received no advanced information about the air in the brain and its possible side effects. Imagine their concern and anguish during the four days they waited for the patient to wake after surgery! If they had been warned of the possibility and realized that it is not uncommon, their level of concern could have been minimized. This is yet another example of why it pays to interview more than one neurosurgeon and always ask questions of your care team throughout the DBS process.

Chapter Sixteen
Hospital Hints for Care Partners

The following list offers hints for care partners or any family member or friend who may be waiting at the hospital during surgery:

- Know *approximately* how long the surgery will last. Of course, things may go more quickly than expected, or there may be issues that slow down the surgeon, but the neurosurgeon or one of his or her nurses should be able to estimate the time for you.

- It's not necessary to wait at the hospital for the entire time surgery is taking place. If you have a cell phone, you can leave that number with the staff at the desk in the family waiting area. Someone will call you if there is anything to report while you are out.

- Bring something to keep occupied (e.g., books or magazines, knitting, crossword puzzles), and bring more of it than you think you'll need. *Don't* plan to use the time in the waiting room to call old friends or return work calls. Those would have to be made outside the hospital, because most hospitals do not allow cell-phone use in most areas of facility.

- Bring a buddy or buddies. You can keep each other company and take turns waiting while the other goes to get lunch, etc.

- Don't overdo the number of buddies, however. Having the entire extended family there at the hospital will be stressful for everyone involved, and it can be disruptive for hospital staff and other patients.

• Have a system prepared in advance for notification of other friends and family members. Are you going to do a "phone tree," where everyone is responsible for calling at least one other person on a list? Are you going to send out e-mails?

> For keeping friends and family up-to-date, we used a service called FamilyLink; for a very reasonable fee ($4.95 per day, as of October 31, 2008), it allows you to create a list ahead of time of up to thirty phone numbers. Then, whoever you choose can record a message of any length that will be sent to everyone on your list. You can send as many messages per day as you want for the same daily fee. This service was a godsend because it meant that Paul only had to make one call. He didn't have to remember who he'd reached and who he hadn't, or what information he'd already relayed to whom—very helpful when you are exhausted and anxious. To learn more about FamilyLink, go to http://www.familylinkusa.com/information/faq.html, contact Tom Zawistowski at TomZ@FamilyLinkUSA.com or call (800)846-4630. I am sure that there are other companies that provide a similar service.

• Choose someone in whom you can confide. This may be someone who is with you at the hospital, or it might be a friend 1000 miles away. Sitting through hours of surgery, not knowing what the outcome will be or if there will be complications, etc., is very stressful. Care partners need to take care of themselves, too.

• Leave the hospital occasionally. Go home or to your hotel room and take a bubble bath. Go shopping. Take a nap.

Choosing Your Support People for Surgery

> Sometimes our mates are not the best people to have with us at the hospital. It is important to talk ahead of time about what you expect from your care partner and what that person should expect to do.
> Some patients (me, for example) like the comfort of knowing that someone is always with them in case they need something. Others want to be left alone; they'll ring the call

button if they need something.

Many care partners feel that if they aren't always doing something for the patient, they are not doing their job. When put in situations where there is nothing they can do, such as when you are in the recovery room after surgery, they may need to go for a walk, go shopping (my husband left to buy hair clippers), do laundry or do something active so that they can deal with feeling powerless.

Some care partners may not have as much empathy as we'd like. If they think that pain medication is for sissies, you might want someone else. It is important to have someone who will respond to your needs.

Chapter Seventeen
Surgery #1—Implanting the Leads

Procedures may differ somewhat from one neurosurgeon to another, but I will describe how my surgery went. (I have spoken to others who told me that their experiences were similar.)

You will most likely come into the hospital the night before your surgery. This way, your lab work can be checked one more time, and the neurosurgeon can be sure that you don't have food, fluids, or medication before the surgery. (You may be allowed to take non-Parkinson's medications.) Many surgeons don't schedule more than one DBS surgery per day because there is no way of being certain how long the procedure will take. Personally, I would not want a neurosurgeon who performs more than one surgery per day to operate on me. I would be worried about his becoming fatigued or that he might rush the operation in order to get on to the next patient. However, I am not a medical professional, and there may be technological breakthroughs or team approaches being used that would affect the surgical process. If you surgeon makes a compelling case for doing multiple operations per day, it is up to you to decide how you feel about that.

On the morning of the surgery, you will be awakened very early (that's assuming that you got any sleep in the first place). My nurse came in around 5:30 a.m. to get me prepped for surgery. You may be asked to shower with antimicrobial soap and shampoo to reduce the possibility of infection.

Some surgeons require that the entire head be shaved; others only shave the areas in which they will be working. Areas that are shaved are swabbed with antimicrobial solution. Next, a stereotactic frame, or "halo," may be attached to your head—the frame is anchored (screwed) at four points on the skull: just past the outer edge of each eyebrow and at the corresponding two points at the back of your skull. These areas are numbed before the screws are placed, and you may also receive anti-anxiety medication to relax you. In my case, I didn't feel any pain with the placement of the halo, although I did feel a slight pressure.

Some surgeons use a "frameless" technology when they perform

DBS, so you might not have the experience of having a halo attached.

You may be required to say "See you later" to your family prior to the placement of the frame. I saw my family after the placement, however, as I was being wheeled to the operating room.

A nurse will most likely check to make sure that you are the correct patient and to confirm the procedure that will be performed. Then you will go into the operating room.

It seems that some neurosurgeons use only local anesthetic to make the single burr hole in the skull for unilateral DBS (or two holes for bilateral systems). I was very glad that I was lightly sedated for that part of the procedure. If you are nervous about this part of the procedure, ask your neurosurgeon if light sedation is possible.

Magnetic resonance imaging (MRI) and CT scans are used to assist the surgical team with the lead placement. I do not remember any of that part of the procedure, but I do recall being awake for the lead placement.

You need to be awake for the lead implantation so that you can give the team feedback and help them to know when they have the lead in the right place. In addition to confirming that the lead is on target, standard neurological tests, such as finger-tapping or counting backwards, are used to rule out effects such as impaired limb movement, severe speech impacts, etc.

Once one lead is placed, you can go back to sleep. If you are only having one "side" done, you may be finished with the surgery, or your neurosurgeon may choose to implant the neurostimulator, since you are there anyway. If you are having bilateral surgery, you will be sedated again while one side is sutured and the other side is prepared.

Although each person's brain is unique and should be treated that way, the surgery commonly takes three to six hours *per side*. My neurosurgeon gave me the choice of stopping after the first side, in case I had had enough of being bolted to the table. I chose to continue, but it was comforting to know that I had the option to stop. My bilateral surgery took about seven and a half hours. (A more detailed account comes later in this chapter.)

I had considerable head and neck pain for a couple of weeks after surgery because of the "tunneling" done for wire placement in my scalp and neck, but although this pain is normal, it is not *common*. In other words, my pain did not indicate that something had gone wrong with the operation, which is what I feared. Most patients, however, do not seem to experience such pain.

The following three entries, written by Paul, give you a bit of the flavor of how a care partner might be feeling during and immediately after the procedure. It is so interesting now to read his thoughts at the time. I have also added my own recollection of the surgery.

Surgical Progress
Wednesday, January 25, 2006

Hi—husband Paul here. Jackie stayed in the hospital overnight last night. This morning, Rosemary (Jackie's mom) and I were there to see her before the process started. At 7:15, she was wheeled to a prep room, where all of her hair was shaved off. We agreed that she has a nicely shaped scalp and may want to go with this "look." They made us leave while they numbed her skin in four places and attached the "halo" by screwing pointy bolts into those numbed places. Afterward, she had what she referred to as her "Hannibal Lecter" look—the titanium frame encircled her head at about ear-level. She said it didn't hurt, but it felt tight. After that, we parted ways, and she is in the OR. We got updates when she was prepped, when the doctor entered the OR, and the latest was that the wire was in on the right side of her brain, and she was awake, doing tests.

They did the right side first because that lobe controls the left side of the body. She has been most affected on the left side.

Bless you all for your calls and prayers of support. I'm going back to the waiting area now. Four more hours or so, and she'll be wired!

~*~

First Surgery Done
Wednesday, January 25, 2006

Hi

She is out of surgery and in recovery. Everything went fine. We'll get to see her in about an hour. More later ...

Paul

~*~

The Endless, Exhausted Waiting
Thursday, January 26, 2006

Hi

Jackie had an uneventful night, unless you count the nursing events—they woke her up every hour, understandable in this post-surgical context. However, they woke her every two hours the night before her surgery. No need to check vital signs pre-surgery. I know I'm venting, but why is there so little resting allowed in your hospital bed? This happens every hospital visit. Okay, got that off my chest. What it adds up to is that she is impossibly tired. Other than that, she is feeling better. There is still considerable pain, but the medications are controlling it. She's eating a little, too.

She is still in the post-operative ICU, although she had the doctor's blessing to move to a regular room five hours ago. Rosemary has been with her this morning while I did laundry. Heading back over there now.

Thank you all for your support!

Paul

~*~

My side of the story
Sunday, January 24, 2006

The night before the surgery, I checked into the hospital at around 4:30 p.m. I was given a supper tray, but I don't remember eating much.

I was supposed to try to rest. The doctor on duty said that he would make a note on my chart to do my lab work and vitals "late," so that I could get some sleep. He also gave me a little extra Ativan to help with my anxiety. I tried to do the relaxation exercise from *Prepare for Surgery, Heal Faster* with mixed results. I took my last dose of Sinemet at 10 p.m.

At around 10:30 or so, I think I finally dozed off. I was rudely awakened at 2:00 a.m. for my lab work and then again at 4:00 a.m. for vital signs. Finally, at about 5:00 a.m., I was told that Dr. Rezai's nurse, Ellen Dooling, would be coming to get me shortly. Paul and Mom came in to officially say "see you later," although they did come along to watch the "shearing."

It was about 5:45 a.m. when Ellen shaved my head and put on the stereotactic frame, also known as a "halo." I didn't have any pain as the halo went on. I had intended for Paul to take photos, but we both forgot. I did have him save a piece of my hair. (I had given my hairdresser free rein on the last haircut before the surgery, and he had chosen to color my hair as well as cut it. I liked that color and wanted him to be able to duplicate it.)

It was time to say good-bye again to Mom and Paul and go off to have another CT scan. That was uneventful. I gave Ellen two music CDs as we briefly parted ways (I would see her in the operating room.)

I remember a long gurney ride and then being "parked" in a room with four curtained stalls. Mine was the only bed there. I remember a nurse checking my wristband to confirm who I was and the type of procedure I was having. Then an anesthesiologist came in to ask, for the umpteenth time, if I had ever had any problems with anesthesia. No.

I vaguely remember meeting a couple of the nurses and being asked to take some deep breaths.

The next thing I knew, I was awake and feeling pain at one of the sites where the stereotactic frame was bolted to my head. I asked for and received more local anesthetic. I could hear a staticky sound, like a radio tuned between the stations. I could hear Dr. Cooper and Dr. Rezai talking, and out of the corner of my left eye, I could see an image projected onto the wall. It looked like a wire going into an image of my brain.

I asked Dr. Cooper a couple of questions, which seemed to annoy him. He seemed to be waiting for the static sound to disappear, which would indicate that he was in the right spot with the probe. Along the way, as he moved the probe millimeters at a time, I had to do what I call "party tricks" (the movements in a typical neurological exam).

I was very thirsty, but I couldn't have anything to drink, not even ice chips to wet my mouth. Dr. Rezai offered me a sponge to suck on, which tasted about like I imagine a kitchen sponge would taste. The next time I requested something wet, I got what seemed to be lemon lip gloss. It didn't help much with the mouth dryness, but it tasted better than the sponge!

The next thing I knew, I heard the Indigo Girls singing "Closer to Fine." I opened my eyes and heard a man say, "I like your music. Who is this singing?" I smiled and asked what was happening. "We're almost done," he said.

When I woke up, my head felt as if it was full of stinging bees. I was very surprised, because none of the people I knew who had already had DBS surgery mentioned anything about pain!

I remember getting both fentanyl by injection and Percocet by mouth and thinking, "My God, this should be enough to numb a horse!" but the combination of the two made my pain just bearable.

I tried to sleep, but between the incredible pain and the nurse who woke me up every hour (probably to make sure that the large dose of painkillers hadn't killed me), I wasn't getting much rest.

I was in a small room with glass walls that were covered with curtains on two sides. It turned out that this was a room within the recovery area. When I was coherent enough to ask (which was late morning, the day after the surgery), I was told that I would be staying there until a bed in a regular room opened up. My surgery had been done on a Wednesday, and Wednesdays were the biggest days for surgeries at Cleveland Clinic.

When Sierra came to see me, she seemed surprised that I was having so much pain but said that it wasn't unheard of.

That evening, Dr. Rezai came in with an entourage: Ellen and two or three men. One I recognized as the anesthesiologist who had said he liked my OR music. They were also surprised to hear about my pain. Dr. Rezai asked if there was anything he could do for me. I offhandedly remarked that I could use some peace and quiet (my roommate had her three adult children and several grandchildren arrive with a carload of McDonald's food and were settling in to stay for a few hours).

Dr. Rezai said, "I'll see what I can do," and within an hour, I had been moved! My insurance wouldn't cover a private room, but my new roommate had just come out of the recovery room and was heavily medicated.

I realized during the room transfer that in spite of the pain, I could move more smoothly than I would have expected. That felt great!

I spent one more night in the hospital (for a total of three). I was discharged with a prescription for Percocet and instructions to call the neurology resident on call if my pain got worse, if I noticed redness or swelling around the stitches, or if I ran a fever above 101°.

Paul and Mom took me back to the hotel. (We had rented a one-bedroom suite for the ten days that we were going to be in town. We chose a hotel right on the Cleveland Clinic campus, even though it was outrageously expensive.) I napped a little and felt pretty good for awhile.

It was during this lull that I convinced Mom and Paul that I felt well enough to go out and celebrate. Unfortunately, by the time we looked on Citysearch.com for restaurants, agreed on one, and Paul thought he had figured out how to get there, I wasn't feeling so well anymore. Although the Chinese restaurant that we finally found had the best General Tso's chicken I've ever had, my head was really throbbing, and we had to leave early. I think it was due to being upright for a couple of hours, letting my pain medication wear off, and getting jarred whenever Paul would drive over one of Cleveland's plentiful potholes.

Mom had to fly back home the next morning, so Paul took her to the airport while I slept. I wasn't feeling too bad, so I didn't take the Percocet on schedule. Boy, was that a mistake! The pain came back with a vengeance.

We ended up going to the emergency room because I was convinced that something was wrong. Everything was fine, but I was given more painkillers and told to keep taking them every four to six hours for the next few days.

I would spend that whole weekend in a Percocet-induced fog. My routine was "Eat a little. Take two pills. Go to sleep. Repeat." I remember thinking, "Yikes. If I'm in this much pain now, what the heck is it going to be like when I have the pacemakers in my chest?"

Photo 1:

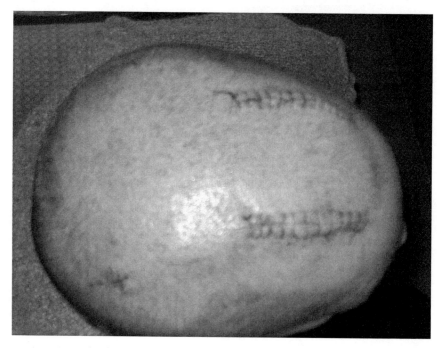

The view of my incisions, from the top of my head. Three of the four incisions are visible in this photo.

Photo 2:

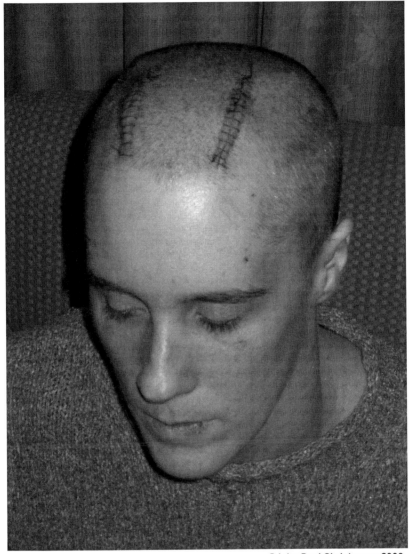

Showing off my "racing stripes" two days after brain surgery.

Chapter Eighteen
Surgery #2—Neurostimulator Implantation

Many surgeons choose to do the implantation of the neurostimulator in a separate surgery, particularly if you are having bilateral leads implanted.

During this surgery, the neurostimulator is placed in a "pocket" that the surgeon creates from muscle tissue and anchors it to the chest wall. Usually, it is near the sternum and below the collar bone. Depending on the surgeon's personal preference, your physical structure, and the condition of your skin, the surgeon may use glue and/or stitches to close the wound.

The extension wires are attached on one end to the neurostimulator and then the other end is threaded under the skin, up behind the ear, where it is hooked up by a connector to the lead wires.

Although the procedure is done under general anesthetic, it is often an outpatient operation. In other words, you don't stay overnight at the hospital. Note that this may change, based on your own personal health status, your doctor's or insurance company's preference, or if there are complications with the procedure. My surgery involved placement of two neurotransmitters and took about three to three and a half hours.

Photo 3:

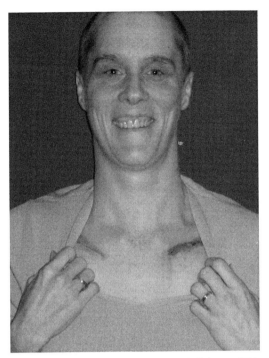

These are incisions from my neurostimulators. My surgeon used surgical glue to close the wounds, and there was less scarring. Depending on the location of your neurostimulators, the condition of your skin, and other factors, your surgeon may be able to use glue, too. When I had one neurostimulator moved in July 2006 because it got rubbed by my seatbelt when I was driving, the surgeon had to use stitches.

My recollections of the neurotransmitter-installation surgery experience
Monday, January 30, 2006

On Sunday night, Paul drove to the airport to pick up my friend, Kari. She and I had gone to high school together. We had lost touch over the years, but I had heard that she was working on a nursing degree. When she heard about my upcoming surgery (you can't keep anything a secret in my hometown of fewer than 4,000 people), she asked if there was anything she could do to help. So I asked her to come down for the second surgery and drive back to Minneapolis with us. I had figured that by that point, Paul would be ready for a break!

On Monday, January 30, Dr. Rezai was going to put in the two neurostimulators during an outpatient procedure. It was scheduled to take about three hours and was supposed to start around 11 a.m. As with the previous surgery, I had been told that I couldn't have any food or medication after midnight Sunday. I managed to get permission to take my first dose of Sinemet, as usual, and also my Wellbutrin, but by noon, when I would have had another half of a Sinemet 25/100, I was starting to get dyskinetic.

I had been asked for a urine specimen when I first was put into a waiting room. Because I hadn't had any liquid to speak of since the night before, I was unable to "produce." The nurse who had originally put me in the room told me not to worry about it. However, a new nurse came on at 11 a.m., and by 12:30, she was really on my case about providing them with some pee. Of course, now the pressure was on, so I really couldn't go. Then it occurred to me that they were waiting for the urine to be certain that I wasn't pregnant. So I asked, and that was indeed the case. I explained that I had had my tubes tied but to no avail.

Finally, I could pee enough to give them the sample that they needed. This moved the process along considerably, and I believe I headed for the operating room around 2:15 p.m. This time, there was a much shorter gurney ride to what I assumed was the same pre-op room. After that, I really don't remember anything until awakening with great pain and dyskinesia in the recovery room. I was also freezing!

I lay there for who knows how long, waiting until the anesthesia wore off enough so that I could ask my nurse for another blanket and some Sinemet. She brought me more pain medication, a nice warm blanket, and some ice chips for my sore throat (from the breathing tube that was inserted for general anesthetic). However, when I asked for the Sinemet, the nurse frowned, saying "Oh, I'm sorry. That medication hasn't been ordered."

"I really need that medication!" I implored. "This was Parkinson's-related surgery. I can't believe it wasn't ordered!"

"I can order it now, but it will take awhile," the nurse said. "Do you have any with you?"

This struck me as a very stupid question, since all I was wearing was a hospital gown. Where would I put medication? She then asked if my husband might have some.

I knew that Paul was supposed to have a stash of my Sinemet with him, so I asked the nurse to call him. She reached him, but it took him about forty-five minutes to arrive. By then, I was extremely dyskinetic and furious with Paul for taking so long. He had been out doing laundry and hadn't had the Sinemet with him, so he'd had to go to our hotel to get it.

Once I got the Sinemet, my dyskinesia stopped. While I continued to recover from the anesthetic, I listened to Paul and Kari speak with awe as they looked at the CT scans on the light box behind my head. Apparently, there were scans of my head that showed the placement of the leads in my brain and scans of my neck and chest that showed the neurostimulators. Paul and Kari both said they felt like they were looking at scans of the "Bionic Woman."

I've never gotten to see those scans, but since then, I really have felt like I can do almost anything again.

Occasionally, there are reasons for the surgeon to place the neurotransmitter in the abdomen instead of the upper chest. I have heard from a couple of patients who have had this placement. They report that clothing waistbands and lap seatbelts may constrict the neurotransmitter, depending on the exact abdominal placement of the unit. Patients also report that they can sometimes feel the neurotransmitter when they bend over. It is not painful, just unnerving the first few times one notices it.

Most patients with whom I spoke said that they had at least some pain associated with this surgery. Although it may be difficult to follow your post-operative lifting instructions, it really is important to try to avoid lifting your arms above your head for the first few days. General post-op instructions say to avoid lifting anything ten pounds or heavier for four weeks. (This is another reason why having help around the house after your surgery is critical.)

Things to Make Post-Op More Pleasant

• Ice packs. These were suggested by Northwest Parkinson's Foundation executive director Bill Bell, who used them on his mother when she had DBS. Paul couldn't find the old-fashioned ice packs that one fills with ice cubes, and we didn't have access to a freezer to use the blue-ice ones. We had to use the blue vinyl gloves (I hate vinyl because of its damaging environmental impacts) filled with ice. I looked like I had blue cow udders sprouting from my head! The ice, however, really helped with the pain and possibly kept down the swelling of my scalp. We also put icepacks, wrapped in a towel, on my neurostimulator sites.

• I-pod/MP3 player/CD player with headphones and the soothing, relaxing music of your choice. Your care partner should hold on to this when you are not using it so that it doesn't get stolen or lost. Hospitals are very noisy places, and rest is an important part of the healing process. Anything you can do to ensure peace and quiet will help.

• Ear plugs. For muffling all of those hospital noises when you are trying to sleep.

• List of phone numbers of family and friends. Even if you have them memorized now, chances are good that for the first few hours or days after the surgery, you will not be able to remember them.

• Clothing with a loose-fitting collar. I learned this the hard way. Since my surgery was in January in the Midwest, I packed turtlenecks. Not very smart! Getting them over my head was painful. Also, don't put wool clothing in direct contact with your skin. It will make your incisions itch a lot!

• Small towel to put between you and your vehicle's seat belt. When you leave the hospital or clinic after having the neurostimulators installed, your chest will be sore on one or both sides. If there is a stimulator on your left side, depending on its location and your height, the shoulder belt may go right across your incision. Ouch! Using some padding will ease the pain.

Chapter Nineteen
After You Leave the Hospital

Our bodies are all different, so each of us will have a slightly different response to the surgeries involved in DBS. As I've said, no one else I knew who'd had DBS surgery mentioned that they'd had any pain. Yet I had excruciating pain in my head and neck for nearly three weeks after the lead implantation. Because no one I knew had experienced pain, I was concerned that something was wrong. It wasn't. In my informal survey of fifty-eight patients, about half of them reported some level of post-operative pain.

Even if your surgeries go wonderfully and you have no pain whatsoever, you will still need to do a few things to ensure that you stay healthy.

- Follow all of the recommendations on your hospital discharge papers. Make sure that your care partner has a copy.

- Keep your incisions/stitches clean and dry. Use bandages only if specified in your discharge papers.

- Don't do too much too soon. I know a guy who was shooting baskets with his son one day after surgery. He later conceded that this was not the best idea.

- Even though you may feel great, remember that you have incisions that need to stay closed and heal. You also need to limit the amount of weight you lift, per your discharge instructions. This will allow the incisions from the pacemaker surgery to heal.

- If you have been prescribed pain medication and are having pain, take the medication on schedule, whether you need it or not, for the first few days post-op. This will ensure that the pain doesn't get out of control. I can say from experience that this is very important.

• Continue to take your medications for your health condition (PD, ET, or dystonia), as directed by your doctor. Cut down or eliminate medicines only when your doctor tells you to do so! This is very important! Yes, it is true that *some* people—very few, as I understand it—do get to go off their medications for a while after surgery. Good for them! Your doctor will let you know if he or she thinks you are one of those lucky people.

• You may experience varying degrees of confusion for up to a month post-op. The brain swells as a result of the surgical intrusion, and confusion is one side effect. As the swelling subsides, so should the confusion.

Although I denied it vehemently at the time, in retrospect I know that I experienced some confusion and slowed thinking for the first couple of weeks after the brain surgery.

DAZED AND CONFUSED
Friday, January 27, 2006

I was finally moved to a regular hospital room at about 3 p.m. The first thing that my nurse did was a neurological exam (you know the one: "Squeeze my fingers as tightly as you can"; "Don't let me push your legs toward your body"; "Follow the light from my flashlight with your eyes"; etc.). She asked me my name, what day it was, where I was—I did fine. Then she asked me, "Who is president of the United States right now?" I could not, for the life of me, come up with an answer. It took me probably one full minute before I could say "George W. Bush." Maybe my subconscious had been trying to block out that reality.

Next thing I knew, there was a short, birdlike woman at the foot of my bed. She looked really familiar but I couldn't place her. "Do you know who I am?" she asked.

"Yes," I said, but I was lying. Only when I looked at the name on her badge did I realize that it was Sierra. Even then, I couldn't remember exactly what her job was.

She asked if I felt confused, and I replied that no, I really didn't think I was all that confused. (In retrospect, I know that I was.)

My husband also noted that simple decision making was a long process during that time. He would ask me a question like "Do you want me to make you some lunch?" and it would take me several seconds to decide, and then several more seconds to verbalize my decision.

"HOW DOES MY HAIR LOOK?" A FEW WORDS ABOUT HAIR GROWTH

One of the questions that I am asked nearly every time I talk about DBS, either in public or one-on-one, is "How quickly does your hair grow back?" I may get asked this question more often than other women who've had the surgery because I tend to keep my hair pretty short. This is not due to slow growth following surgery; I simply prefer no-maintenance short hair.

Of course, it will depend on how quickly your hair generally grows, and whether your head is completely shaved or the surgeon merely shaves "racing stripes" into your hair to get access to the necessary parts of your brain. In general, though, you will probably have some good "peach fuzz" going within a week or two of the lead placement. I had my surgery at the end of January and had my first haircut in mid-April.

Photo 4

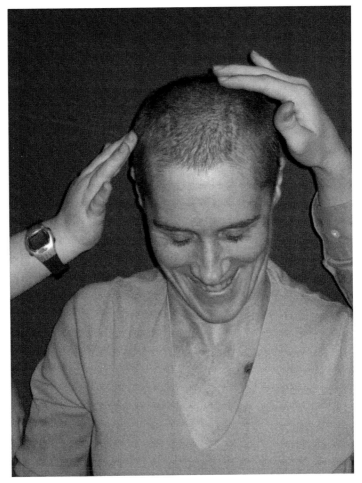

My sons really liked my hair when it was this short. They enjoyed rubbing the stubble. Their efforts to convince me to keep it that short failed, however.

Your head will not be smooth. There will be one or two lumps (depending on whether your surgery is unilateral or bilateral) near the front of your head on top. On men who are balding or who wear their hair *really* short, these may look like the buds of horns.

SOMETHING TO PUT IN YOUR WALLET

When you leave the hospital, you will most likely be given a temporary identification card that says "I have an implanted medical device that may set off your airport/security system" in several languages. You will need this for air travel and at many museums and government buildings, especially in Washington, DC. Later, you will receive a plastic wallet card with the same message. It will also include your device's model, serial number and implantation date, your neurosurgeon's name and phone number, and a phone number for the device manufacturer that you can call if you have any questions or problems. I use this phone number whenever I am scheduled to have a new medical or dental procedure. That way, I can find out if I need to take any special precautions, such as turning my neurostimulators off, or if I need to avoid it altogether.

Chapter Twenty
Expectations vs. Reality

It's important that you and your family discuss everyone's expectations for the outcome of DBS with your surgeon. Ideally, he or she will let you know whether those expectations are realistic. But the moment the system is turned on for the first time and there is any improvement in your symptoms, I believe a whole new set of expectations are created—or if not expectations, then hopes or wishes.

I have been extremely blessed and have had excellent results from my surgery and programming. One particularly poignant moment for me occurred at our **young-onset Parkinson's disease** support group. A new couple had joined the group, and when it was time to split into care partners and Parkies, the care partner told Paul that she had thought *he* was the one with Parkinson's, not me!

Sometimes, an hour or two passes before my body reminds me that I have PD. This is an exquisite feeling, one that I wish everyone who had DBS could experience. But I need to be careful, as does anyone who has had DBS, that I am not lulled into a false sense of security about my health. DBS does not treat all of the symptoms of PD, nor does it stop the progression of the disease.

As you improve over the first six months to one year after your surgery, and you are able to resume many activities you'd had to give up, remind yourself and your family that you still need to take care of yourself. Eat a healthy diet, get plenty of sleep and exercise, and attend a support group. (Many communities are creating groups made up solely of DBS patients and their care partners.)

I know that all of us with PD wish that we could do more to help our care partner, and DBS may be a way to allow us to do that. We need to be realistic, however, and careful about what we take on.

Since I had two procedures (first one side, and the other six years later), the results differed. My initial problem was tremor and the DBS made it disappear. The second side was done

Unfortunately, not everyone gets the results that I received. In fact, one recent study by clinicians at the University of Florida analyzed data from two movement disorder clinics—the University of Florida Movement Disorders, and Beth Israel Movement Disorders Center. The team included nationally renowned neurosurgeons and movement disorder specialists.

They evaluated forty-one patients who came to the clinics because they believed they were not receiving the optimal benefit from DBS surgery. Here is a quick summary of the examination:

- Numerous patients had been misdiagnosed.
- 73 percent of patients had seen a movement disorders specialist before DBS surgery.
- 34 percent were known to have had neuropsychological testing; 10 percent did not have the testing; and in 56 percent of the cases, they were unable to determine whether the patient had been tested.
- 12 percent hadn't tried all of their medication options before choosing surgery.
- 12 percent had "significant cognitive dysfunction" before surgery.

Many of these patients had surgical complications or hardware issues.

- 46 percent of patients had "suboptimally placed leads," which means the neurosurgeon didn't get the lead in the best location to control the patient's symptoms.
- 17 percent needed electrodes replaced.
- 3 patients had "dead" batteries in their neurostimulators.
- 2 patients had infections.
- 1 patient had a broken lead.

Inadequate programming was also a problem. This isn't surprising, considering the lack of specific training requirements for programmers.

- 17 of patients had no access to programming or had difficulties getting to a programmer.

• 37 percent of patients "were inadequately programmed and improved *significantly* [emphasis added] with reprogramming."
• 15 percent had received inadequate programming and experienced "partial improvement" when reprogrammed.
• 51 percent didn't improve despite "extensive reprogramming."

The team also found that 73 percent of patients improved after medication changes. This point underscores the fact that most patients do not go off all medication after surgery. All medication changes should be done in consultation with your doctor.

When all was said and done, 51 percent of the patients who had begun the study with the feeling that the surgery had "failed" eventually got good results.

If you would like to know more, I highly recommend reading the entire article, "Management of Referred Deep Brain Stimulation Failures: A Retrospective Analysis from Two Movement Disorders Centers" by Michael S. Okun, et al. *Archives of Neurology.* 2005:62.

It is my personal belief that this study underscores my suggestions about carefully choosing both your neurosurgeon and your programmer.

Chapter Twenty One
The "Honeymoon" Period

Many patients experience what is known as a **"honeymoon period"** after their lead implantation. Often, there is swelling in the brain that occurs because of all the poking around that your surgeon has been doing in there.

This can result in abatement or decrease in at least some symptoms *without the stimulation turned on.* I was lucky enough to have a honeymoon of nearly three weeks, during which I had almost no dyskinesia, and my rigidity was much less. *It is important to note that, per my doctor's orders, I was still taking my pre-surgery dosages of medications.*

Remember; always call your neurologist if you feel like you don't need your medications. He or she can help you to find out how much or how little you can take and how to reach that dosage safely. Some medications are long-acting, which can result in a crash after about three days if you have under-medicated yourself. Stopping any medication abruptly is never a good idea, unless it's on the advice of your doctor. You never know when the honeymoon will end, but when it does, falls and anxiety are common until you resume medication.

I know others who have not had any honeymoon period and have still had very good results with their surgery, so there appears to be no correlation between the two.

Chapter Twenty Two
"Tune in, Turn On"—The Day You've Been Waiting For

Whether it is five days after your surgery or five weeks, the day on which your deep brain stimulation system is turned on is the big one. (Note: The neurosurgeon does turn on the system and test it during surgery, but it is generally not left on.) This is an excellent indicator of what is reasonable to expect when *your system settings are optimized*. This does not mean that the moment the system is turned on, you will immediately be able to sprint a 100-yard dash.

Of course, there is the usual disclaimer: "Results may vary." But if you could repair an engine or do woodworking or crochet during that "on" time, chances are good that you will be able to do that activity—and probably for a longer period—when the system is on.

Expect to spend the whole day at the clinic or doctor's office. Much of your time will be spent with the programmer as she or he checks the settings on each of the electrodes on each lead. The rest of the time will be spent waiting to see how your body responds.

For initial programming (and often for subsequent sessions), you will be asked to come in "off meds." In other words, you will not take your medication for at least twelve hours before your appointment. The programmer wants to see the effects of the stimulation alone.

Like most visits to the neurologist, you will be asked to do the basic tasks in the standard neurological exam. Then the programmer will program the neurostimulator(s). You will repeat the "party tricks," and the programmer may adjust the voltage again. Usually, you will be asked to wait at the clinic or hospital for an hour or two, to watch for side effects.

Most people report that they do not feel anything when the neurostimulator is turned on or the voltage increased, unless the programmer is establishing the maximum threshold they can tolerate. In this case, they may grimace or feel their muscles contort. I felt a millisecond "zing" run through my body when my programmer first turned on the neurostimulator. I felt my tongue curl when she tried a maximum setting. In general, though, I do not feel any sensation from the system when it is functioning properly.

The Big Day!
Wednesday, March 1, 2006

I wish that we had brought a video camera to film the "before" and "after." I highly recommend that, if you can.

I remember Sierra using what looked like a smaller version of the tracking machines that UPS or FedEx drivers carry. It had a pen or stylus that she used to tap on the screen. Connected to it via a cable was something about the size of a hockey puck. She placed the "puck" over one stimulator at a time. I could feel a very quick (fraction of a second) "zing" sensation as she increased the voltage up to 3.0 volts on each side.

Then she had me do all the "party tricks"—tapping my thumb and forefinger on each hand, touching my forefinger to my nose and back, walking down the hallway, etc.

As I walked down the office hallway and turned to come back, I could hear my husband, Paul, say "It's just like watching the old [pre-PD] Jackie!" As I got closer, I saw that he had tears in his eyes.

Sierra seemed very pleased and said my initial results looked very good. At that point, I thought we were done and could leave. Sierra said that we couldn't leave the clinic; we would have to stick around for at least a couple of hours to see if I experienced any side effects. I thought that was all b.s.—until about an hour and fifteen minutes later, when I began to have severe dyskinesia.

Sierra said that this was not uncommon and that she would turn the voltage down. We would have to increase it slowly.

She set the right stimulator back to 1.0 volts and the left to 0.8 volts. I was really disappointed. That meant more trips to Cleveland—and more expense—but I was determined to let Sierra finish my initial programming.

The number of visits it takes to reach the right voltage for you will vary, as will the number of volts. One side may be different from the other. Our brains are all different, and as the disease progresses, our needs will change.

It is important to know that your brain will adjust to the voltage *and* that your disease will progress, so you *will* need to have the voltage adjusted. If your programmer questions the need for a change, talk to your neurologist (if he or she is not the programmer) or your surgeon.

A FEW WORDS ABOUT PROGRAMMING

Surgery is only half of the DBS equation; programming is the other half. Your surgeon can place the leads in the most perfect spots for your brain, and if the programmer doesn't know what he or she is doing, you will not receive the optimum benefits from the system. Conversely, if your surgeon doesn't get the placement right, the most skilled programmer in the world will not be able to give you optimum results. This is why it pays to shop around.

Recently, Medtronic introduced its "Programming in a Box" concept. This is the description on their website.

On-site programming training

This training is held in a private practitioner's office or in an academic clinic setting, and offers observation of patients and discussion of their motor responses as their Activa Therapy is programmed. Participants receive a minimum of six hours of training, which includes hands-on programming as well as didactic training using Medtronic Neurological's Programming in a Box resource. (Medtronic3, 2008)

This is a start, but there are no federally mandated training requirements for programmers: no licensure requirements, no test to prove that they understand how the system works. Some programmers are neurologists. Many are nurses. A significant number of programmers do it only part-time because their hospital or clinic has not done enough of the surgeries yet to merit a full-time staff person.

This past winter, I was interviewed by some researchers from Japan as part of a DBS study they are doing. I asked the neurosurgeon on the team about programming there. He said that about 95 percent of the programming is done by the neurosurgeons. The other 5 percent is done by neurologists. In Japan, it is almost unheard of for someone other than an MD to program DBS patients.

As the surgery becomes more common and patients learn that they can expect more from the DBS system, I hope that a certification program can be put in place. Unfortunately, due to the significant variability in programmer credentials, the patient advocacy groups may have to be the driving force for better oversight and certification requirements to apply electricity to a person's brain.

In the meantime, if you want to see if there are other programmers in your area, or if you have questions about expectations of programming, you can go to a website called DBS Programmer.com (www.dbsprogrammer. com), which was created and personally funded by a DBS programmer/ advocate for patients. You can register free of charge and check the database for programmers in your area. Programmers can provide as much (or as little) information about their training as they choose, but obviously, those who include more detail are more likely to be contacted. Patients can also request e-mail updates as changes to the database occur.

Tips for Programming Visits

• Always bring someone with you. That person can keep you entertained, and he or she may notice side effects that you don't. If you do have trouble, someone will be there to help.

• You may find that you are tired after a programming session, so plan time for a nap. This is another reason to bring someone along with you.

If you need to travel to have your programming done, always plan on staying overnight, and don't plan to leave before noon the next day. Your programmer may want to adjust the voltage one day and see you again the next day, to determine whether more fine-tuning is necessary.

• Report any side effects or changes to your programmer right away, no matter how small or insignificant they may seem. After one programming visit, I felt my tongue wiggling around in my mouth constantly. It was annoying, but I didn't immediately connect it with the change in voltage. I happened to mention it the following month, and my programmer said, "You should have told me. I can probably fix that." And she did.

• Ask questions and expect logical answers in language that you can understand. Be an informed patient. After all, it's your body that this system is affecting, and it's your time and money being used for the appointment.

• You may be asked to come in for programming off-medications overnight. This allows the programmer to assess what stimulation can do without the help of your medications. Being off-medication also gives the programmer symptoms that can aid the search for the best electrodes. For instance, rigidity or tremor greatly improves when using the best electrode.

PROGRAMMING IS AN ONGOING PROCESS

Very few people find that the setting that is programmed at the first visit is ideal. Most require multiple visits to find a setting that works best. In my informal survey, thirty-eight of the fifty-six people (67.9 percent) who answered the question indicated that one session had not been enough. For me, it took six programming sessions, about a month apart, before my programmer felt that the settings were optimized. This meant five more trips to Cleveland after the initial session, which was expensive and time-consuming, but I felt it was important to let the staff there finish their work.

Once the settings are optimized, it may take six months to a year to get the full benefits of that programming. This can be a time when people fall a lot more. It is possible that this falling is related to the surgery, but many physicians theorize that it happens because patients are trying to do things that they haven't been able to do for a long time. I know that I have certainly tried doing things that I hadn't enjoyed for many years, such as riding a bicycle. I even played a bit in my sixth-grade son's parent/student soccer game!

Your brain will adapt to the new settings, so you will eventually need to have additional adjustments. There is no set timetable for this. For me, when I notice that I am starting to have some dyskinesia and/or my medication is starting to wear off earlier, I know it is time to have an adjustment made. I schedule an appointment with the programmer, and we talk about what my symptoms are. She then makes a change in the voltage and tells me to stay near the clinic (in the waiting room or in the building) for an hour or so, in case I have any problems.

More than half (58 percent) of the people I surveyed said that they had two to four "maintenance" adjustments per year. A much smaller number (14 percent) said that they needed six or more.

DBS is not a cure—at least not for Parkinson's disease—and the disease will progress.

No one knows how long the device will be effective, but patients who have had the system for ten years report that they are still experiencing benefits from it.

"Hey, Baby. What's Your Setting?" Knowing Your Voltage

I have heard from several people living with DBS systems that their programmer is or has been unwilling to let them know the parameters of their neurostimulators. Although this has never been a problem for me, it simply makes no sense.

I am fairly certain that keeping such information from the patient is a violation of the Health Insurance Portability and Accountability Act of 1996 (HIPAA—pronounced "*hip*-uh"). Doctors are allowed to keep information from you if they believe that knowing that information could endanger you or a loved one. I cannot think of a scenario, however, in which it would be dangerous for a patient to know his or her programmed settings.

Remember, too, that everyone is different. Our individual body chemistries and anatomies work with our own DBS systems to create an environment in which some settings will work better than others. The 4.0 volts that keep you functioning without tremor or dystonia would have me jumping around like a marionette being controlled by a hyperactive demon-child, whereas my 3.2 and 3.5 volt settings might not be enough to stop your tremors.

Always ask for a printout of your settings and changes. Your stimulation settings are just like medication doses; you need a record for yourself in case you need to know what your settings are in a hurry. For instance, if you need to have surgery, someone will have to change your settings/turn off the neurostimulators. You will want to make sure that you are put back on the right settings.

Chapter Twenty Three
The Particulars of Programming

Note: If you are an engineer, you may want to skip this chapter. We have attempted to simplify things for the rest of the world, who are not engineers.

Sierra Farris, PA-C, an advocate for patients and a programmer at the Booth Gardner Parkinson Center, Evergreen Hospital, Kirkland, Washington, wrote the bulk of this chapter, which I adapted for inclusion in the book. Any mistakes in the definitions and description of programming are mine alone (although she did review my text.) Sierra has programmed more than 500 DBS patients, as of June 1, 2008, although these are not all people with PD.

Even before I developed PD, I did not understand physics. My last memorable educational encounter with physics was as a high school junior, when the class convinced our teacher to let us study the physics principles displayed by a Slinky.

The goal of this chapter is to help people who are considering deep brain stimulation or who are living with DBS to understand what happens inside their bodies and brain and to provide insight into what goes through the mind of their programmer.

Sierra Farris told me she wishes that every medical professional doing programming would take into consideration the courage and commitment required to undergo a procedure that involves being implanted with wires, batteries, electrodes, and circuit boards. A good programmer respects the patient's awareness of his or her body and involves the patient in the process. A patient who understands the programming process may be able to provide feedback to assist the clinician in finding the best settings. She said that a patient once said to her, "If I [could] buy one of those programmers, I could work through thousands of combinations to find just the right one."

I hope that after you read this chapter, you will come to the conclusion that there are a few combinations that provide good symptomatic relief without causing side effects, and a lot of program settings may not relieve symptoms or may cause adverse side effects—or both. Sierra said that when she speaks to programmers, she tell them, "Always listen to your patients. They tell you what you need to know, even when you can't see it or feel it yourself."

> *"The brain is a magnificent tangle of connections of emotion, experience, and intuition that [is] beyond the reach of human understanding."* ~ Sierra Farris, PA-C

BASIC PARAMETERS OF ELECTROPHYSIOLOGY AND NEUROSTIMULATION

When I was gathering information for this chapter, Sierra told me that her goal as a programmer is "to design a field of stimulation that improves symptoms as much as possible, while avoiding side effects. Once the neurosurgeon puts the hardware in place, I need to work with it where it is." (In some cases, leads may be moved to a new location, which involves another surgery. More on that in another chapter.)

Programmers can change three different parameters within the system: voltage (volts), **pulse width** (microseconds), and **frequency** (hertz). Those parameters can be applied to one or more electrode. The electrodes are turned off or on by the clinician or programmer.

MAKING A CIRCUIT

Now we make a mental trip back to elementary school science class, when we messed around with batteries or stuck wires into potatoes. We learned back then that if an electrode is turned on, it must be set as either negative or positive. We must have a negative electrode (cathode) and a positive electrode (anode) to complete an electrical circuit.

In a DBS system, the electrode serving as the cathode is the one that improves your symptoms. The cathode attracts the anode, which, in turn, spawns negative electrons in search of a positive. The field or area of stimulation is determined by which electrode is turned on as the negative and which electrode is turned on as the positive electrode.

Ideally, programmers only use the electrodes they need to produce the best benefits from stimulation and with the fewest side effects. Remember, not all electrodes are actually in the brain target, and more is not always better. The important point here is that electrode selection can determine whether benefit is gained and whether side effects get in the way of optimal stimulation. Your programmer will need to be adept at electrode selection.

Otherwise, you may have to endure many programming sessions until the lucky combination is selected. Turning on *all* the electrodes may cause side effects and drain your neurostimulator battery faster. But again, I believe that programmers should have the patient's best interests in mind.

I also feel strongly that the patient should be informed and involved in programming decisions, especially ones that may lead to earlier battery replacement because of high stimulation settings.

Once the appropriate electrode is selected, the programmer can focus on the other possible parameters.

Sierra's List of Key Programming Concepts

Voltage is measured in volts. Although many things have changed since that high school physics class, Ohm's law (voltage is equal to resistance multiplied by current) is still in effect.

Voltage is not unlimited, however. If voltage expands the area of stimulation beyond the target, side effects on your hands, legs, or speech will result. A clinician worth her (or his) salt will know how much is too much. Too little voltage will not fully improve your symptoms. Too much can cause side effects and also possible improvement in symptoms. It is important for you to learn how much voltage you can tolerate without experiencing side effects. Your maximal voltage is established by the accuracy of the neurosurgeon's placement of the lead wire in your brain and the programmer's skill in selection of the electrodes. Voltage seems to play a pivotal role in whether or not motor symptoms are improved.

Pulse width is possibly one of the most overused parameters when encountering stimulation side effects. Each electrical pulsation from your neurostimulator has a duration that is defined by the clinician. Pulse width is measured in microseconds and can be turned up exponentially from 60 to 450. The longer the pulse duration, the stronger the field of stimulation In general terms, however, stronger is not always better. Side effects occur, and the programmer may choose to decrease voltage. If voltage is sacrificed in order to increase pulse width, there is a chance that the benefits to the patient also will be sacrificed.

Frequency is the last parameter the programmer can

change. Frequency is simply defined as the "number of pulses occurring in one second." It is measured in hertz. Clinically used ranges are from 130 hertz to 185 hertz. Frequencies less than 130 have not been found to be as beneficial for the FDA-approved brain targets (STN, GPi, and thalamus).

Frequency is currently (no pun intended) the most amazing and least understood parameter. Programmers know from clinical experience that frequency does matter, and each brain target has a minimal frequency threshold necessary to obtain benefit. Because the topic is very complex and needs more data, however, I will not attempt to explain this programming parameter any further. Patients who are interested (and who have engineering backgrounds) can ask their programmers for occasional literature updates on frequency.

Precision is essential in DBS, for both the neurosurgeon and the programmer. If the electrode is in the wrong place, a programmer will have a difficult time eliciting good results. However, perfect placement of the electrodes can be rendered ineffective by programming mistakes.

When Sierra was explaining programming to me, she put it this way:

The thought of all of these variables can be daunting to a programmer. This may translate into many visits for the patient to achieve the right setting. Or the clinician may use the "shot in the dark" approach by choosing a random setting and expecting the patient to live with it. I think, however, that there is some middle ground. After all, one or two electrodes typically are in the desired target. This quickly eliminates some of the trial and error.

Maximal voltage is important and should not be overshadowed by pulse width. There should be "give and take" between the two to optimize symptom control. However, side effects should not be considered acceptable. If side effects limit benefit, we typically reexamine the field or area of stimulation.

This brings us to monopolar and bipolar polarity options. Polarity determines the size and shape of the area of stimulation. The lead wire is described as quadripolar, which means there are four electrodes that can be activated.

Monopolar polarity indicates that only negative electrodes are turned on and the neurostimulator battery is considered the positive electrode or cathode. Bipolar polarity indicates that both a negative and positive electrode are turned on. Remember, the clinician can make any of the electrodes negative or positive and in any combination.

Monopolar stimulation creates a field or area of stimulation that extends in all directions away from the negative electrode, kind of like a balloon shape. Depending on the voltage and pulse width, this can be quite a large area of stimulation. Bipolar stimulation is used when more control is desired, most often to avoid side effects as the area of stimulation is more contained.

(See Figures 2 and 3 to get a "picture" of how it works.)

Figure 5

MONOPOLAR STIMULATION

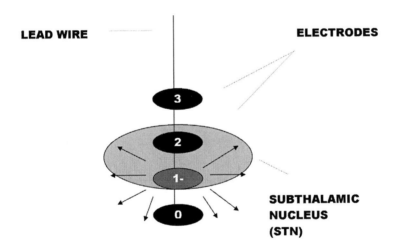

LEAD WIRE

ELECTRODES

SUBTHALAMIC
NUCLEUS
(STN)

BIPOLAR STIMULATION

Figure 6

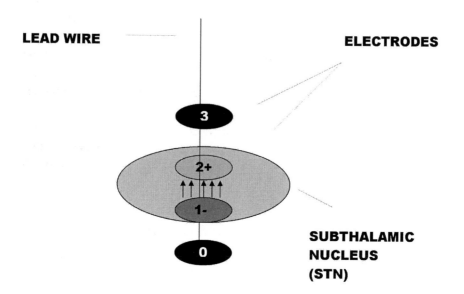

LEAD WIRE

ELECTRODES

SUBTHALAMIC NUCLEUS (STN)

Graphic by Jackie Hunt Christensen

MONOPOLAR OR BIPOLAR? THAT IS THE QUESTION

There is no general, correct answer. What works will vary from patient to patient. Sierra told me that she has found that using bipolar stimulation can be helpful if DBS-induced dyskinesia is a problem, because it helps contain the area of stimulation from spreading too far, potentially causing side effects.

When using monopolar stimulation, there is not a positive electrode turned on—the neurostimulator battery functions as the positive—so stimulation spreads in all directions. Monopolar stimulation can be very powerful and some patients will need that power to control their symptoms. Monopolar settings, however, can easily cause side effects if the stimulation settings are too high. The tradeoff is that the patient may need less voltage overall, which would prolong battery life. The bottom line is that programmers should use what is best for the patient with the goal of improving symptoms, without causing side effects.

Sierra recommends that at each appointment, your programmer should check your DBS system to make sure that the wires are intact and that the battery life is adequate. (See Chapter 27, "Should I Buy Jumper Cables? Do You Need Battery Replacement?")

Troubleshooting

If the electrical circuit is intact and at least one electrode on the lead wire is in the target of the brain, the DBS system should relieve at least some of your motor symptoms (remember your best "on" time). However, any mechanical device can malfunction. It is not always easy to determine when or if the system is broken. X-rays may be required and even then, they are not always helpful. The patient typically knows when something is wrong and, in Sierra's experience, is usually the most accurate indicator of a problem. Occasionally, however, the patient doesn't associate a change in symptoms with a possible device malfunction. I know a couple of people who had broken wires for more than a year before the problem was discovered. This makes routine system checks by your programmer even more important.

- A breakdown in the silicone covering of the wire can allow stimulation to escape and cause disconcerting but predictable symptoms, such as tingling, muscle spasms, crawling sensations, or shocks. A break in the wire can result in similar symptoms, in addition to a return of the symptoms that DBS was supposed to improve.

•A break in the wire can cause a short circuit. This can lead to several undesirable problems, including wearing down the battery rapidly, heating the wire and its silicone coating; stimulation side effects that you hadn't previously experienced; and loss of symptom control for your PD.

• Damaged wires can be replaced, but that replacement involves surgery and thus should not be done unless other non-invasive ways to fix the problem have been unsuccessful. This will be covered more in Chapter 24, "'Care and Feeding' of Your DBS System."

Sierra had some final remarks on the subject of programming that she asked me to include. I think they are a good way to end this chapter.

You chose DBS because you reached a point where your symptoms were controlling your life. You have gone through a lot of pain, time, and money to get to that point. You deserve the best possible chance of success and the best possible outcome. Think of your programmer as your employee, because in a sense, he is. A good programmer is able to determine your best stimulation settings, because he or she has a good understanding of the topics in this chapter, as well as a really good understanding of the health condition being treated, the medications, disease progression, and the individual who is living with all the above. If you don't "click" with your clinician, move on and find someone else.

Chapter Twenty Four
"Care and Feeding" of Your DBS System

Even though most of us are more interested in the things that DBS will allow us to *do*, there are still a few activities or situations that should be done with extra care or avoided altogether. Most of them have to do with proximity to **electromagnetic interference (EMI).** In its literature for medical professionals about DBS, Medtronic describes EMI as:

… a field of energy (electric, magnetic, or a combination of both) generated by equipment found in the home, work, medical, or public environments that is strong enough to interfere with neurostimulator function. Neurostimulators include features that provide protection from electromagnetic interference. Most electrical devices and magnets encountered in a normal day are unlikely to affect the operation of a neurostimulator. However, strong sources of electromagnetic interference can result in the following:

- **Serious injury or death,** resulting from heating of the implanted neurostimulation system components, which can damage surrounding tissue
- **System damage,** requiring surgical replacement or result in a loss of or change in symptom control
- **Operational changes to the neurostimulator,** causing it to switch ON or OFF, or to reset to default factory settings, which may result in loss of stimulation, return of symptoms, and require reprogramming by the physician
- **Unexpected changes in stimulation,** causing a momentary increase in stimulation or intermittent stimulation, which some patients have described as "shocking" or "jolting." Although the unexpected change in stimulation may feel uncomfortable, it does not cause damage or injury. In rare cases, as a result of the unexpected stimulation, patients have fallen down and been injured (Medtronic, 2002).

You should be able to do most of the things that you did prior to surgery, but here are some tools and household appliances we need to use with care—they contain magnets or motors that could turn off the Activa device. I have put the information into a grid to that you can make photocopies to post in your home or office or take to an appointment with a health-care provider.

ACTIVITIES AND SITUATIONS THAT REQUIRE PRECAUTIONS OR SHOULD BE AVOIDED

In this increasingly wireless world, there will constantly be new products and new sources of electromagnetic interference being added. The list below is not meant to be exhaustive; rather, it's to give you a list of the types of equipment and environments that can cause problems.

Figure 7

Relative Safety
of Various EMI Sources

Safe to use if tool or appliance is kept at least 4"/10 cm away from stimulators	Avoid/use with extreme caution	Consult Medtronic patient care representative for safety parameters
Refrigerator/freezer -- don't lean against magnetic strip on open edge of door*	Antenna of citizen band (CB) radio or ham radio*	Bone growth regulators*
Storm door -- don't lean against magnetic strip on open edge of door*	Electric induction heaters used in industry to bend plastic*	Dental drills and ultrasonic probes*
AM/FM radios*	Resistance welders*	Diagnostic ultrasound
Conventional wired phones, cordless phones, cellular phones*	Electric arc welding equipment	Electrolysis*
Car radios/speakers -- keep away from chest when carrying/lifting*	Electric steel furnaces*	Hyperbaric chambers*
Home stereo speakers -- keep away from chest when carrying/lifting*	High voltage (safe if outside the fenced area)*	Other implanted devices (e.g., defibrillators, pacemakers, cochlear implants)*
Sewing machine -- avoid close proximity to motor*	High power amateur transmitters*	Laser procedures*
Salon hair dryer -- avoid close proximity to motor*	Linear power amplifiers*	Radiation therapy*
Power tools -- also keep away from leads and extensions. Be particularly careful if equipment would become dangerous if your symptoms were to return (e.g., bandsaw, power drill)*	Microwave communication transmitters (safe if outside the fenced area)*	TENS (transcutaneous external neurostimulator) units*
Computer hard drive -- if repairing, keep your chest/upper body at least 4"/10 cm from your work*	Television and radio transmitting towers (safe if outside the fenced area)*	Mammography or other X-rays requiring tight enclosure*
MP3 players/Ipods#	Perfusion systems*	
Be sure to carry your patient programmer with you so that you can check to see whether your system is on or to turn it on/off.	Magnets or other equipment that generates strong magnetic fields*	
	Magnetic degaussers*	

Figure 8

Relative Safety
of Various EMI Sources

The following are believed to be safe and do not require special precautions.*	Avoid/use with extreme caution	The following are considered unsafe or require special precautions because they may cause harm to the system or the patient, not merely turn the neurostimulator ON/OFF
CT or CAT (computerized axial tomography) scans*	Therapeutic magnets (blankets, mattresses, joint wraps) -- keep at least 10 "/25 cm away from neurostimulators	Defibrillators/cardioversion*
Diagnostic X-rays/fluoroscopy* (see exceptions for mammography/other tight-enclosure X-rays)	Security gates* -- see special instructions	Diathermy
Magnetoencephalography (MEG)*	Theft detection systems* -- see special instructions	Electrocautery*
PET (positition emission tomography) scans*	Magnetic clip-on sunglasses#	High-output ultrasonics/lithotripsy*
	Invisible fencing for pets#	MRI (magnetic resonance imaging)
	Electronic gaming systems (e.g., Wii, Xbox 360, Playstation 3) with wireless controllers; Nintendo DS in wireless mode#	
	Hand-held charting devices used in hospitals and clinics#	
	Nextel phone/2-way radio combination#	
	Baby monitors, especially the base#	
	Ultrasonic toothbrushes#	

* from Medtronic, 2002

from anecdotal information gathered from other DBS patients and/or programmers

Dealing with Security Gates and Theft-Detection Systems

It is virtually impossible to go anywhere in America without encountering some sort of security or theft-detection system that could turn off your device. It runs the gamut, from the obvious airport metal detectors and security gates to visible theft-detection systems in retail stores to unseen surveillance systems in hotels and other buildings. It is best to avoid these systems, when possible.

At the airport

When checking in for your flight, ask a ticket agent or airport employee whether you need to go to a specific security checkpoint for screening. For example, you may be asked to go to the checkpoint that airport employees use. When you reach the checkpoint, tell the Transportation Safety Administration (TSA) employee that you have a pacemaker. (Don't try to explain a neurostimulator. For TSA's concerns, it is a pacemaker.) He or she may ask to see your Medtronic or ANS ID card, although I have only been asked to show my card at one airport—in San Francisco. In most cases, you will go through the security line and when you reach the point where you would go through the metal detector, you tell the TSA agent that you have a pacemaker. He or she will direct you as to where to go next (sometimes you wait in a chair next to the screening machine; other times you may be directed to an area off to the side) until another TSA agent can do a "pat-down." The agent will use his or her hands on the various areas of your body, rather than using a metal-detection wand. Your belongings will go through the screening machine like everyone else's.

In government buildings

The procedure is similar to that of an airport. The main differences are that you are much more likely to need to show your device ID card, and you may not have to undergo a full pat-down.

In retail stores, libraries, or places with visible security systems

If there is a security guard present, inform him or her of your situation and ask if it is possible to have a hand-search done instead of going through the gates. If it is possible to walk around the outer side of the system, that is ideal. This can often be done at libraries. If you need to go through the device, try to walk through the center of the threshold. Getting too close to either pedestal may turn off your neurostimulator. If there is only one pedestal, walk as far away from it as possible.

Physical Activities to Do with Care or to Avoid

Medtronic warns against any activities "that include sudden, excessive, or repetitive bending, twisting, bouncing, or stretching"[1] because of concerns that you could damage the system. They are particularly concerned about activities that involve twisting or stretching of your neck because the movements might break, bend, or dislodge an extension wire. The result would be that your system would apply stimulation to the breakage point instead of applying it to your brain (ouch!), work intermittently or not at all, or drain the battery. It would also mean that you would have to have surgery to repair or replace the component. So, one could infer that activities like aerobics, Pilates, tai chi, and yoga should be done with care. Playing football or rugby, wrestling, or bungee-jumping are probably all bad ideas.

You also need to avoid activities that could cause the components of the system to heat up, thereby potentially damaging the surrounding tissue in your body, as well as harming the system itself. Activities that fall into this category include using hot tubs with a water temperature above 98 degrees, saunas, or steam rooms.

Your head needs to be protected from injury, too. If you are going to Rollerblade, ride a bicycle, or drive or ride on a motorcycle, be sure to wear a well-fitting helmet.

People who have undergone DBS surgery should not scuba dive below thirty-three feet because the pressure could damage the system.

Individual Experiences with EMI

These guidelines should protect *most* people who have had DBS, but just as some people are more sensitive than others to medications, foods, or the sun, some DBS patients find themselves much more affected by ambient levels of EMI.

If your system does get turned on or off by something, you can report it at the Food and Drug Administration's (FDA) "MedWatch" website. Just go to http://www.fda.gov/medwatch/report/consumer/consumer.htm, and click on the "Online Reporting Form" link. By reporting such incidents, you will help to build evidence of this problem and, I hope, elicit some changes to protect patients from this phenomenon.

Chapter Twenty Five
The Annual Maintenance Check

Like the battery/batteries in your car or your camera or your smoke detector, your DBS pacemaker batteries will eventually lose power and need to be replaced. However, unlike your car and camera, which have warning lights to let you know that battery failure is imminent, or your smoke detector, which beeps when the battery is low, the DBS systems available today have no uniform advance way of telling you it is replacement time.

Your programmer can do a battery and wire check in just a few minutes. Think of this as a "50,000-mile tune-up," although it is probably a good idea for her to do this, as well as check your impedances, any time you have any programming changed. This checkup will most likely become more important to do as you and the DBS system age. No one knows how the hardware components will hold up beyond a ten-year period.

Photo 5

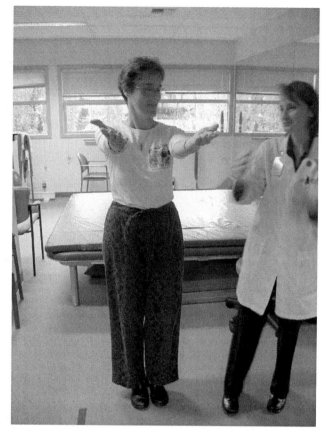

Sierra Farris, PA-C, has me do some of the parts of a standard neurological examination before making any adjustments to my neurostimulators' settings. I had not taken any Parkinson's medications for more than 12 hours, per Sierra's request.

Photo 6

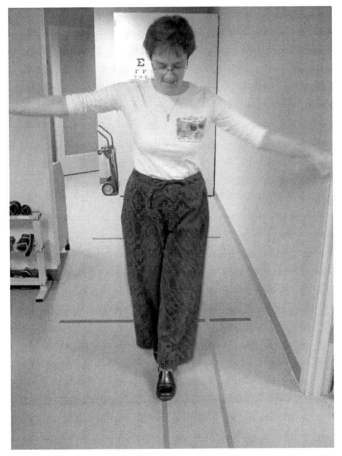

I "walk the line" after 12 hours without medication.

Photo 7

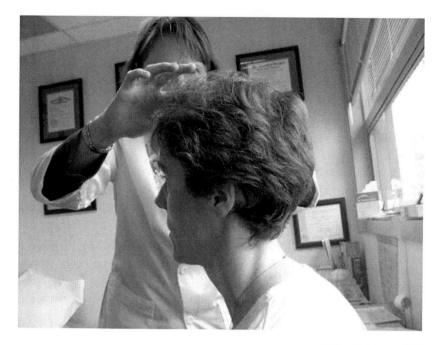

Sierra checks the path of each lead and extension to make sure there is no skin thinning or erosion. .

Photo 8

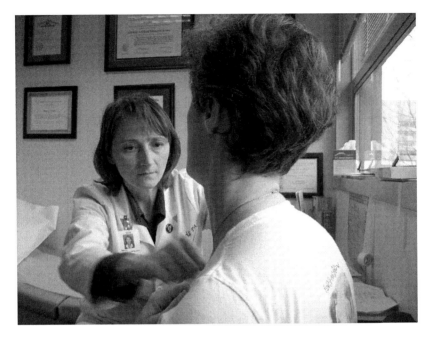

Sierra places the programming device over my right neurostimulator in preparation for a change in voltage. The device must be directly over the neurostimulator for the change to take effect. **Most patients do not feel anything when programming changes are made. A few people report a momentary tingle.**

Photo 9

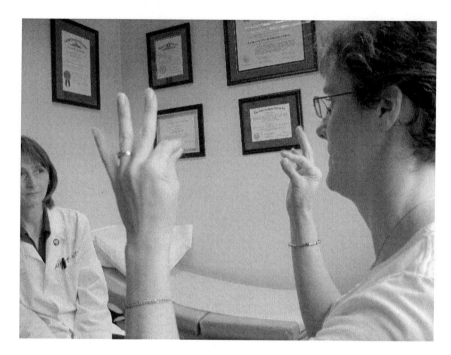

Sierra has made some programming changes and is having me do "party tricks" (more tasks from the standard neurological exam) to assess the effects.

Chapter Twenty Six
Long-Term Side Effects of DBS Surgery

Since DBS has only been in existence for about twenty years and available with insurance/Medicare approval since 2001, data on its long-term effects are sparse. We have no idea whether there is any impact on living with this device system in our bodies for thirty years or more, but the same holds true for most of the medications used to treat Parkinson's disease.

There are some data that suggest that the following conditions may occur in some patients after DBS surgery:

> • Depression (either worsening of previous depression or a new case in someone who had not previously experienced it)

> • Anxiety (same as above)

> • Changes in speech, particularly low volume, slurred speech, and speech articulation (DBS-STN.org, 2006). These effects may not appear immediately. Changes may be in voice volume or in speech quality, or both.

> • Weight gain of at least ten to fifteen pounds within the first year of surgery

> • Obsessive-compulsive behavior and/or addictive behavior (such as gambling, shopping, etc.), other personality changes

> • Changes in sleep patterns (Research has found that some people sleep better after DBS surgery; others do not.)

The reasons for weight gain are easy to surmise. For those with PD or ET, reducing or eliminating tremor or dyskinesia means you are not constantly moving and burning calories.

Speech changes may be a result of disease progression or DBS surgery. Regardless of the cause, these changes are very frustrating for the patient and those around her.

SOME WAYS TO DEAL WITH VOICE CHANGES

• Use yoga or breathing exercises to make sure that you have adequate air. (Have you ever noticed how difficult it is to speak when you've had to get to the phone that was ringing in the next room?)

• Get speech therapy, such as Lee Silverman Voice Therapy (LSVT), or others.

• "Think 'loud'!" This is the motto of the Lee Silverman Voice Therapy program (www.lsvt.org). All it means is that when we speak, we should imagine ourselves doing it *loudly*! Then, if we're lucky, it should be just loud enough for conversation.

• Sing along with the car radio or stereo in your house. Read aloud to your care partner, kids, grandkids. Volunteer to read aloud for children's story hour at your local library. Ask for feedback. Urge others to politely tell you when you need to speak louder. (Note that this doesn't necessarily work with children, especially teenagers. They may prefer to hang on to their "I couldn't hear you" excuse to avoid chores, curfews, etc.)

• Get an analog sound meter—the kind in which a needle goes up or down in reaction to sounds—at a Radio Shack or other store that sells audio equipment. Practice speaking so that your voice stays in the green range.

HARDWARE PROBLEMS THAT MAY OCCUR

There are a couple of things that very occasionally go wrong with DBS systems. Wire breakage or damage is the most common. The insulated wiring used in deep brain stimulation systems is approximately the diameter of a piece of spaghetti, so it is possible to envision that over months and years of use, it could break completely or develop tiny fractures in the insulating material. Also, as mentioned earlier, high heat could affect the integrity of the silicone insulation.

Things that can potentially put your wiring at risk include repeated instances of reaching for things high above your head; fast, sudden movements of your head and neck (some, if not all, chiropractic manipulations of your head and neck must become a thing of the past); and blows to the head at one of the wiring sites. This one may seem unlikely, but you would be surprised! Many people with PD report that Parkinson's disease has affected their spatial skills so we find ourselves misjudging the width or height of doorways and other openings.

February 2008
Reflecting on My Own Experience with Hardware Problems

Last November, I suddenly began experiencing dyskinesia again on my left side. This was a very unwelcome recurrence and was especially disconcerting because it was occurring only on one side. My "garage door opener" (technically, it's called the Access Review Controller or Access Therapy Controller), which allows me to determine whether or not a neurostimulator is on or off and to change the mode to on or off) indicated that my stimulators were on. Around this same time, I notice that sometimes I experienced a buzzing/tingling sensation in my left ear. It also occurred in my left hand and foot, although with much less frequency. The two symptoms got me worrying that perhaps I had broken a wire.

113

The first thing I did was to contact my local programmer to have her do a wire check. She verified that both neurostimulators were on. Luckily, I asked her to write down the settings for each one. Later that day, I e-mailed my initial programmer, whom I had seen in October. When she compared the parameters that she had set to those recorded by my local programmer, there had been a significant change in my settings.

Sierra, my initial programmer, said that she suspected that one of the wires might be damaged. She said that a series of very specialized x-rays would need to be taken to see if this was the case.

She helped me to get an appointment with my neurosurgeon back in Cleveland. To make a long story shorter, I went back to Cleveland Clinic. The programmer there said that the neurostimulator on the right side of my chest, which controls the left side of my body, had reverted back to factory settings. This was the cause of my dyskinesia. She reprogrammed it, and the symptoms subsided. When I met with Dr. Rezai, I expressed concern about the tingling. He said that he wanted to see if the tingling went away after my body adjusted to the reprogramming. He emphasized that he didn't want to put me through surgery unless it was necessary because of the health risks inherent with any surgery. He told me to keep him posted on the ear tingling. If it continued, he would go back in to examine the wire to the neurostimulator first and then the lead to the brain. Thus, I returned to Minneapolis for the holidays, without dyskinesia but with continued tingling in my left ear.

I happened to see my neurologist at a holiday event and mentioned the trip to Cleveland. The next business day, my local programmer called to say that she had informed a Medtronic engineer of my symptoms and suggested that I call her. I did, and she said she had seen similar problems in other patients. She claimed that the connector behind the ear was typically the problem and that it could be taken apart, cleaned out, and reassembled in about twenty minutes. The procedure could even be done with just a local anesthetic!

While I was glad to hear that the surgery wasn't a big deal, I did not want to be awake for this remodeling project! I did decide that since the procedure was allegedly simple, that I would not travel all the way to Cleveland to have it done.

I was able to get on the schedule of a neurosurgeon at the University of Minnesota. Their policy for procedures like this includes a night in the hospital to receive twenty-four hours of intravenous antibiotics.

Once again, I chose the month of January to have surgery. (You would think I'd learn). I went in at about 10 a.m. on a day that was absolutely frigid. I don't think that the temperature was supposed to rise above 0° F. I'll explain later why this is relevant.

I still do not understand how this happened, but we had to wait for an operating room until after 3 p.m. The neurosurgeon then explained that it might be necessary to replace more than just the connector, depending on how the components south of the connector checked out. This would include the wire from the connector to the neurostimulator and the neurostimulator itself. My husband and I were quite surprised at this, but there didn't seem to be any other way to find out, other than the surgery. The neurosurgeon wrote "This Side" in black Sharpie marker and made arrows pointing up toward my ear and down toward the neurostimulator.

When I woke up a couple of hours later, my chest hurt so I knew that something in my chest had been replaced. I remember asking for my Sinemet, which of course had not been ordered. Then I asked to see my husband and was told I had to wait until I was moved to a regular room. And why was I not in a regular room yet? Apparently, I was not breathing enough and the recovery room nurses were not going to let me out of their sight until I took more than ten breaths per minute. I was convinced I was ready to go, so I focused all of my attention on my breathing and within fifteen minutes, I was deemed fit to leave.

When I got up to my room and saw my husband, he said that the connector, neurostimulator, and connecting wire on the left side had been replaced. Apparently, the circuit to one of the electrodes was faulty.

Now I was glad for the night in the hospital because it meant stronger pain medication, which I needed for the chest incision. That one hurt much more than the one behind my ear. Fortunately, the surgeon was able to use the same pocket of muscle tissue to place the new neurostimulator. Otherwise, I would have been really sore!

Leaving the hospital the next evening was particularly painful because the temperature outside was still below 0°, and I couldn't stop shivering. The moral of this story is "Be ready for anything—and avoid having surgery in the winter, if you live in a cold climate."

Some DBS patients have reported "**lead migration**." In other words, the lead wire was surgically placed in one spot but something—perhaps repeated stretching or other movements—caused the electrode(s) to be out of range of the stimulation target. When this happens, the lead wire needs to be moved and placed again. Of course, this means going through the first stage of the surgery all over again. Lead migration could occur at any time, once the leads have been implanted.

Erosion is another long-term hardware complication that can occur. This means that the skin over the neurostimulator or over the capped wires on top of the head becomes thin and can rip open. Infection can develop quickly, so it is important to report this to your doctor immediately if you notice any scabs or wounds on or near any part of your DBS system. Sometimes the wound can be stitched closed but often, the wire or neurostimulator needs to be moved. I had my left neurostimulator moved a few months after my initial surgery because the shoulder seat belt in my car rubbed on it whenever I drove my car. I didn't want to take the risk of having the skin erode and tear.

Once again, these potential hardware problems underscore the notion that DBS is not an event. You will presumably be living with these components or their replacements for the rest of your life, so it is in your best interests to ensure that they continue to work properly.

Chapter Twenty Seven
"Should I Buy Jumper Cables?" Do You Need Battery Replacement?

If you have a Kinetra (the larger of the three Medtronic units), your programmer or doctor can get an instant determination of the remaining power in its battery. Members of a DBS e-mail listserve (DBS_surgery on Yahoo.com) report that these units lose power gradually. Some people report that when their batteries begin to run low, they feel lethargic, as if they are "running out of juice."

Soletra and Itrel II users have to rely on symptoms as an indication that the battery is low. You may experience a slight drop in voltage about one month before the battery depletes. If you find tremors returning, the battery in your neurostimulator may be getting low. Your programmer can track the battery charge and how fast it is dropping. This helps to plan when to replace the neurostimulator. Because DBS helps to eliminate the need for at least some of your medication, you should replace the neurostimulator before the battery becomes too low to provide adequate stimulation, consistently and reliably. If your programmer gives you printouts after checkups, you can also track your battery charge or battery voltage. For example, once the Soletra reaches 3.64 volts, the remaining battery charge depletes fast. The rate of depletion depends on your stimulation settings. Your programmer can get an estimate of remaining battery life from Medtronic technical support to help plan for replacement.

Rechargeable batteries are in the works, but there is no word yet as to when they will be widely available. I have asked jokingly if it will mean having to plug myself into a socket or wearing a little solar panel on my head, but apparently neither of those methods is part of the plan for rechargeables at this time.

Chapter Twenty Eight
Alternatives to DBS

If, after reading this and talking with your doctor and others, you decide that DBS is not for you, there are alternatives. The same is true if you have been told that you are not a good surgical candidate.

You can participate in clinical trials. New therapies are tested on small groups of volunteers for effectiveness and safety. For Parkinson's patients, a new trial for Duodopa, an external pump that delivers micro-doses of levodopa in a gel form to the small intestine, looks promising. This system, similar to the insulin pump for diabetics, should avoid side effects, such as dyskinesia, because of the constant administration of very small amounts of levodopa.

Parkinson's patients can learn more about clinical trials that are recruiting by visiting www.PDtrials.org or www.clinicaltrials.gov.

By seeing a movement disorder specialist (MDS) at least once a year, you can make sure that you have access to the latest treatments. Keep seeing your family doctor, if you feel you are getting good care, but because family physicians and even neurologists need to know about so many other diseases and disorders, keeping up with the Parkinson's literature is difficult to fit into their schedules. Add the MDS, too, if you can afford it.

Exercise both your body and your mind. Staying mentally and physically active can help to keep your symptoms from worsening and will also keep you in shape for the next thing that comes along.

You also can explore complementary therapies, such as tai chi and relaxation therapies, to reduce stress, as stress makes symptoms worse. Physical therapy, occupational therapy, and speech therapy help to keep you in the best shape and function possible.

If you are feeling depressed or anxious about your situation, please seek help. It is appropriate to feel depressed and frustrated when a treatment option is not open to you, or if it doesn't work as expected. There are many therapists and support groups available that can help you deal with your feelings.

Chapter Twenty Nine
What If Something Better Comes Along?

Research into treatments for all of the conditions being treated with DBS is ongoing, so eventually, something better *will* come along.

One way to get involved in the quest for better treatments and a cure for Parkinson's disease is to join organizations that are working on those efforts. The Parkinson's Action Network, for instance, represents the public policy voice of the PD community. They educate policymakers and politicians about Parkinson's disease and how it affects our lives, the community and the economy. No previous advocacy experience is necessary; just a desire to rid the world of PD. See the "Resources" section at the end of the book for contact information for Parkinson's Action Network and other PD organizations.

The deep brain stimulation system is intended to be reversible, meaning that it can be turned off—which is easy—and removed—which, depending on how long you have had the system, might not be so easy. Over a period of several months, the leads and extensions become "scarred in," meaning that scar tissue builds up around them. This could make removal very painful.

Part of the reason that I bring this up is that there is a theory about Parkinson's disease which that postulates that the dopamine system is only one of several systems in the brain that is affected. Dr. Heiko Braak of Germany believes that there are six stages to PD (Braak, 2004), and that the substantia nigra, where dopamine is produced, is not affected until stage 3 or 4. Stages 1 and 2 affect the medulla oblongata and the olfactory bulb. Changes in or loss of sense of smell may be related to this stage. Stages 5 and 6 affect the mature neocortex. Some researchers claim that loss of or diminished sense of smell, constipation, and sleep disorders are all part of the early Braak stages. There is evidence that the heart and the gastrointestinal tract may be affected, too.

The Braak theory makes perfect sense to me, but my DBS system only deals with one of the affected parts of the brain. What about the other areas? All I can say is that the current system is controlling the symptoms that were most difficult for me, and I will adapt as needed.

In the meantime, I can use my renewed mobility to raise awareness and funding for better treatments and cures of all of the neurodegenerative diseases.

Bibliography

Braak, H., et al. "Stages in the development of Parkinson's disease pathology," *Cell and Tissue Research*. 2004 Oct, 318(1):121-34.

Diekema, DJ, et al. "Antimicrobial Resistance Trends and Outbreak Frequency in United States Hospitals," *Clinical Infectious Diseases*. 38(2004)78-85.

Friehs, Gerhard M., Catherine Ojakangas, Linda L. Carpenter, Benjamin Greenberg, and Kelvin L. Chou. *Surgical Aspects of Deep Brain Stimulation*. Medicine and Health Rhode Island, Apr 2006. Accessed online at http://findarticles.com/p/articles/mi_qa4100/is_200604/ai_n17182196 on June 10, 2008.

Internal Revenue Service. *Medical and Dental Expenses*. Government publication 502. 2007.

Kaiser Permanente Northern California. *Patient Information about Sub-Thalamic Nucleus (STN) Deep Brain Stimulation*. Clinical Functional Neuroscience Program. Revised 2/2005. Accessed online at http://www. permanente.net/homepage/kaiser/pdf/36020.pdf on July 19, 2007.

Medtronic, Inc. History of Deep Brain Stimulation. 2008. Accessed online at http://www.medtronic.com/physician/activa/history.html on June 10, 2008.

Medtronic, Inc. [Medtronic2] news release. "Medtronic Activa Deep Brain Stimulation Patient Referral Advisor Software Launched in United States." April 16, 2008.

Medtronic, Inc. [Medtronic3] Small Group Training and Patient Services. Accessed online at http://www.medtronic.com/physician/activa/

smlgroup.html on October 31,

Medtronic Patient Services and Technical Services. *Considerations for Patients with a Medtronic Deep Brain Stimulation System for Movement Disorders.* April 2, 2002.

Moore, Samuel K. "Psychiatry's Shocking New Tools, Continued." *IEEE* [Institute of Electrical and Electronics Engineers, Inc.] *Spectrum OnLine.* Accessed online at http://www.spectrum.ieee.org/mar06/3050/4 on June 9, 2008. First published March 2006.

Okun, Michael S, Hubert H. Hernandez, and Kelley D. Foote. *Am I a Candidate for Deep Brain Stimulation? And What Are the Ten Questions I Need to Ask about DBS?* University of Florida Movement Disorders Center website. Accessed online at http://mdc.mbi.ufl.edu/candidate/candidate-intro.htm on October 2, 2007.

Okun, Michael S., *et al.* "Management of Referred Deep Brain Stimulation Failures: A Retrospective Analysis from Two Movement Disorders Centers." *Archives of Neurology.* 62(2005)1251-1255.
Stewart, RJ, JM Desaloms, and MK Sanghera. "Stimulation of the Subthalamic Nucleus for the Treatment of Parkinson's Disease: Postoperative Management, Programming and Rehabilitation." *Journal of Neuroscience Nursing.* 37(2005):108-114.

Glossary

access review contoller/access therapy controller: the patient controller for the DBS system. It looks like a large garage-door opener and can be used to verify the status of the system and the batteries in the controller; turns the DBS system on or off. Kinetra models can vary the voltage within a narrow range.

Activa: brand name for the deep brain stimulation system by Medtronic, Inc.

bilateral stimulation: having lead wires implanted in both sides of the brain to control symptoms in both sides off the body.

bradykinesia: medical term for the slowed movements that often occur with Parkinson's disease.

cognitive dysfunction: problems with mental processes, such as reasoning, perception, learning, decision making; a common symptom of PD that is only beginning to be studied.

dopamine system: the parts of the brain in which dopamine, a chemical in the brain that tells muscles when and how to move. In PD patients, an estimated sixty to eighty percent of the dopamine-producing neurons in the brain are dead or damaged.

dyskinesia: uncontrolled writhing movements that often occur in Parkinson's patients after years of levodopa therapy; much more common in young-onset PD.

dystonia: abnormal tension or tightness of muscle tissue caused by chronic muscle contractions. It may cause jerky movements in the affected limb or part of the body. Dyskinesia is a form of dystonia.

electrode: the contact area at the tip of the lead wire that can emit or receive electrical signals from the neurotransmitter. There are usually four electrodes per lead wire on the Medtronic systems in use in 2008.

electromagnetic interference: energy from other electrical and/or magnetic devices that can interfere with the operation of implanted medical devices, such as neurostimulators, cardiac pacemakers/ and defibrillators.

erosion: when the skin over part of the DBS system becomes thin and breaks open.

extension wire: the piece of insulated wire that connects the lead wire to the neurostimulator.

essential tremor (ET): a neurological disorder that results in tremor (shaking), usually of the hands or head, although affects other parts of the body as well. As with Parkinson's disease, the cause of ET is unknown, and there is no cure at the present time.

frequency: the number of pulses emitted by a neurostimulator in one second; measured in hertz.

globus pallidus interna (GPi): a part of the brain located in the area called the basal ganglia. It is near the substantia nigra (the area depleted of dopamine-producing neurons in PD). It is one of the locations that may be targeted in DBS surgery.

"honeymoon period": an indeterminate period of time that *may* occur between the implantation of leads in the brain and the programming of the neurostimulators, when symptoms lessen or abate. Some patients experience no honeymoon period, while it may last for weeks in others.

impedance: measurement of how electricity travels though a given material. Every tissue has different electrical impedance determined by its molecular composition. [http://www.imaginis.com/t-scan/impedance.asp]

lead: the piece of silicone-insulated wire that is implanted in the brain.

Electrodes are placed at the tip, which is inserted into the target area of the brain.

lead migration: the lead wire moves from its original placement site in the brain.

levodopa: synthetic drug compound that the brain converts to dopamine. Levodopa is used primarily to treat the motor symptoms of Parkinson's disease, although it becomes less effective over time. Sinemet is the brand name for the drug.

motor symptoms: movement-related symptoms of Parkinson's disease, such as tremors or slowed movement

movement disorder specialist: a neurologist who has received additional specialized training in movement disorders, such as essential tremor, Parkinson's disease, Huntington's disease, and muscular dystrophy.

neurostimulator: the part of the deep brain stimulation system responsible for generating electrical impulses (stimulation). It is contained in the same component as the battery that supplies the power to generate the stimulation. The neurostimulator is sometimes also called the pacemaker or the implanted pulse generator (IPG).

neurosurgeon: type of surgeon who specializes in performing operations on the brain or other parts of the nervous system.

nosocomial infection: an infection that is acquired in a hospital.

"on/off time": "on time" describes the period when medication controls the motor symptoms of Parkinson's disease; no side effects (e.g., dyskinesia) are observed. "Off time" refers to the period when symptoms are not controlled and/or medication is not effective. For example, it is possible to have times when you take your medication as usual, but it does not work, and you experience motor symptoms as if you hadn't taken any medication.

pallidotomy: surgical procedure in which permanent lesions (scars) are made on the globus pallidus in the brain, in an attempt to control tremors or muscle rigidity.

Parkinson's disease (PD): chronic progressive neurological disease marked by tremor, muscle rigidity, slowed movement, and/or poor balance, as well as psychological symptoms (depression, changes in cognition, memory, etc.). Its cause is unknown and there is no cure. Deep brain stimulation is one of the most recent attempts to treat the motor symptoms of the disease.

programming: the process of using the various electrodes on a stimulator to find the best combination of electrical impulses from the various electrodes to provide optimal symptom control.

pulse width: the length of time that each electrical pulsation from a neurostimulator occurs, usually from 60–450 microseconds.

stereotactic frame: also called a "halo," this metal frame is attached to the head at four points with screws. Bars on the frame allow it to be attached to the operating table to prevent the patient from moving his or her head during surgery.

sub-thalamic nucleus (STN): an area of the brain that is often targeted to treat the motor symptoms of Parkinson's disease

thalamotomy: surgical procedure in which lesions (scars) are created in the thalamus area in the brain. This operation is intended to control motor symptoms of Parkinson's disease or essential tremor. It is not performed very often anymore because of the risks involved and because DBS has similar effects. DBS is reversible, while thalamatomy and pallidotomy are not.

unilateral stimulation: electrical stimulation of only one side of the brain. Most commonly used in essential tremor or when Parkinson's disease symptoms affect one side predominantly.

voltage: the measurement of "the ability of an electric field to give energy to electric charges." [HowStuffWorks.com]

young-onset Parkinson's disease: When the symptoms of PD are diagnosed before age 50, it is referred to as "young-onset Parkinson's disease" or "early-onset Parkinson's disease."

Resources

Am I a Candidate for Deep Brain Stimulation? And What Are the Ten Questions I Need to Ask about DBS? By Michael S. Okun, M.D., Hubert H. Fernandez, M.D., and Kelly D. Foote, M.D.
http://mdc.mbi.ufl.edu/candidate/candidate-intro.htm

The Parkinson Alliance/The Tuchman Foundation
PO Box 308
Kingston, NJ 08528-0308
Phone: 800-579-8440 or 609-688-0870
Fax: 609-688-0875
Internet: www.parkinsonalliance.org
www.dbs-stn.org
www.dbsprogrammer.com

Margaret Tuchman, president of the Parkinson Alliance, had DBS surgery in 2000 and has been working since that time to educate patients, clinicians, and the public about the procedure and its long-term effects.

National Parkinson Foundation
1501 N.W. 9th Avenue / Bob Hope Road Miami, Florida 33136-1494Telephone: (305) 243-6666Toll Free National: 1-800-327-4545Fax: (305) 243-5595Email: contact@parkinson.org
Internet: www.parkinson.org

The National Parkinson Foundation has a free booklet on DBS. It can be ordered from their website. Their website also has "Ask the Doctor," "Ask the Surgical Team," and "Talk to a Speech Clinician"—features that can be very helpful to people who have had DBS or are contemplating it.

Parkinson's Disease Foundation (Main Office)
1359 Broadway, Suite 1509
New York, NY 10018

Toll-free Helpline: (800) 457-6676
Phone: (212) 923-4700
Fax: (212) 923-4778
Email: info@pdf.org
Internet: www.pdf.org

The Parkinson's Disease Foundation has a free brochure about DBS surgery for PD. It is available on their website under "Publications."

Parkinson's Action Network
1025 Vermont Avenue Northwest, Suite 1120
Washington, DC 20005
Phone: 800-850-4726 or 202-638-4101
Fax: 202-638-7257
Email: info@parkinsonsaction.org
Internet: www.parkinsonsaction.org

The Parkinson's Action Network (PAN) is the unified voice of the Parkinson's disease community—advocating for more than one million Americans and their families.

The Parkinson's Institute and Clinical Center
675 Almanor Avenue
Sunnyvale, CA 94085
Toll-free phone: 1-800-655-2273
Internet: www.thepi.org

"Founded in 1988, The Parkinson's Institute and Clinical Center (PI) is America's only independent non-profit organization that provides basic and clinical research, clinical trials and a comprehensive movement disorder patient clinic for Parkinson's disease (PD) and related neurological movement disorders, all under one roof. Our mission is to find the causes, provide first class patient care and discover a cure. Our unique freestanding organization supports a strong collaboration of translational medicine designed to more directly connect research to patient care – from the "bench to bedside"."

WE MOVE (Worldwide Education and Awareness for Movement Disorders) 204 West 84th Street New York, NY 10024
E-mail: wemove@wemove.org
Internet: www.wemove.org

WE MOVE is "dedicated to educating and informing patients, professionals, and the public about the latest clinical advances, management, and treatment options for neurologic movement disorders." Their website has a searchable database of movement disorder specialists; patients can look for the clinician closest to them, free of charge.

Yahoo! DBS Surgery (online only)
Internet: health.groups.yahoo.com/group/DBSsurgery

"This group is for the discussion of deep brain stimulation surgical procedures. Key words: DBS, Parkinson's disease, essential tremor, dystonia, MS, multiple sclerosis, brain surgery, Medtronic, Activa."

Appendix A: Florida Surgical Questionnaire for Parkinson Disease (FLASQ-PD)

Date of Evaluation: _____

Please verify a diagnosis of idiopathic PD by assuring your patient meets the UK Brain Bank Criteria (Hughs, et. al.):

A. Diagnosis of Idiopathic Parkinson's Disease

Diagnosis 1: Is Bradykinesia present? Yes/No (Please circle response)

Diagnosis 2: *(check if present):*

___ Rigidity (Stiffness in arms, leg, or neck)

___ 4-6 Hertz resting tremor

___ Postural instability not caused by primary visual, vestibular, cerebellar, proprioceptive

dysfunction

Does your patient have at least 2 of the above? Yes/No (Please circle response)

Diagnosis 3: *(check if present):*

___ Unilateral onset

___ Rest tremor present

___ Progressive disorder

___ Persistent asymmetry affecting side of onset most

___ Excellent response (70-100%) to levodopa

___ Severe levodopa induced dyskinesia

___ Levodopa response for 5 years or more

___ Clinical course of 5 years or more

Does your patient have at least 3 of the above? Yes/No (Please circle response)

("Yes" answers to all 3 questions above suggest the diagnosis of idiopathic PD)

B. Findings Suggestive of Parkinsonism Due to a Process Other Than Idiopathic PD

Primitive Reflexes

    1- RED FLAG – presence of a grasp, snout, root, suck, or Myerson's sign

    N/A – not done/unknown

Presence of supranuclear gaze palsy

    1- RED FLAG – supranuclear gaze palsy present

    N/A – not done/unknown

Presence of ideomotor apraxia

    1- RED FLAG – ideomotor apraxia present

    N/A – not done/unknown

Presence of autonomic dysfunction

    1- RED FLAG - presence of new severe orthostatic hypotension not due to medications.

    erectile dysfunction or other autonomic disturbance within the first year or two of disease

    onset

    N/A – not done/unknown

Presence of a wide based gait

    1- RED FLAG – wide based gait present

    N/A – not done/unknown

Presence of more than mild dementia

    1- RED FLAG – frequently disoriented or severe cognitive difficulties or severe memory

    problems, or anomia

    N/A – not done, not known

Presence of severe psychosis

    1- RED FLAG – presence of severe psychosis, refractory to medications

    N/A – not done, not known

History of unresponsiveness to levodopa

    1- RED FLAG- Parkinsonism is clearly not responsive to levodopa, or patient is

    dopamine naïve, or patient has not had a trial of levodopa

    N/A – not done, not known

(Any of the "FLAG's" above may be contraindications to surgery)

C. Patient Characteristics *(Circle the one best answer that characterizes your Parkinson's Disease Surgical Candidate):*

1. Age:

    0 - >80

    1 – 71-80

    2 – 61-70

    3 - <61

2. Duration of Parkinson's symptoms:

    0 - <3 years

    1 – 4-5 years

    2 - >5 years

3. On-Off fluctuations (medications wear off, fluctuate with dyskinesia and akinesia)?

    0 – no

    1 – yes

4. Dyskinesias

    0 – none

    1 - <50% of the time

    2 - >50% of the time

5. Dystonia

    0 – none

    1 - <50% of the time

    2- >50% of the time

General Patient Characteristics Subscore ____

D. Favorable/Unfavorable Characteristics

6. Gait Freezing

    0 – not responsive to levodopa during the best "on"

    1 – responsive to levodopa during the best "on"

    NA – not applicable

7. Postural Instability

    0 – not responsive to levodopa during the best "on"

    1 – responsive to levodopa during the best "on"

    NA – not applicable

8. Warfarin or other blood thinners

    0 – on warfarin or another blood thinner besides antiplatelet therapy

    1 – not on warfarin or another blood thinner besides antiplatelet therapy

9. Cognitive function:

    0 - memory difficulties or frontal deficits

    1 – no signs or symptoms of cognitive dysfunction

10. Swallowing function

    0 – frequent choking or aspiration

    1 - occasional choking

    2 - rare choking

    3 - no swallowing difficulties

11. Continence

0- incontinent of bowel and bladder

1- incontinent of bladder only

2- no incontinence

12. Depression

0 – severe depression with vegetative symptoms

1 – treated, moderate depression

2 – mild depressive symptoms

3 – no depression

13. Psychosis:

0 – frequent hallucinations

1 – occasional hallucinations- probable medication-related

2 – no hallucinations

Favorable/Unfavorable Characteristics Subscore _____

E. Medication Trials *(circle the best answer)*

14. Historical response to levodopa:

0 uncertain historical response to levodopa, or no trial of levodopa

1 – history of modest improvement with levodopa

2 – history of marked improvement with levodopa

15. Trial of Sinemet (Carbidopa/Levodopa or Madopar or equivalent):

0 – No Trial or less than three times a day

1 – Sinemet three times a day

2 – Sinemet four times a day

3 – Sinemet greater than four times a day

16. Trial of Dopamine Agonist:

0 – No Trial or less than three times a day

1 – Dopamine Agonist three times a day

2 – Dopamine Agonist four times a day

3 – Dopamine Agonist greater than four times a day

17. Trial of Sinemet Extender

0 – No Trial

1 - Trial of either tolcapone or entacapone

18. Trial of a combination of sinemet or equivalent with a dopamine agonist

0 – No trial

1 – Trial of sinemet or equivalent with a dopamine agonist

Medication Trial Subscore: _____

FLASQ-PD Scoring:

A. Met Diagnostic Criteria of Idiopathic PD: Yes/No

B. Contraindications (FLAGS) Subscore: _____ (8 possible- any flags=likely not a good candidate)

C. General Characteristics Subscore _____ (10 possible)

D. Favorable/Unfavorable Characteristics Subscore: _____ (14 possible)

E. Medication Trial Subscore _____ (10 possible)

Total Scale Score (C+D+E): _____ (34 possible)

Presence of Refractory Tremor:

Yes/No (Presence of moderate to severe tremor that is refractory to high doses and combinations of levodopa, dopamine agonists, and anticholinergics may be an indication for surgery in some candidates, independent of their score on the remainder of the questionnaire

Appendix B: DBS Survey Results

Because I wanted this book to tell other stories in addition to my own, I decided to put together a survey. I wrote all of the questions myself. Although I have not had training in statistics or polling, two people with previous experience in creating polls or surveys reviewed my document. After making the suggested changes, the following survey was available online for two months. I used word-of-mouth, e-mails to various PD lists and listserves, and notices in PD newsletters to make DBS patients aware of the survey. I received fifty-eight responses. Not everyone answered all of the questions so that is why the response count does not always add up to fifty-eight. The response percentage will add up to 100 percent of those who answered the question.

3. How much time elapsed between when you first started thinking about DBS and when you had the operations?

	Response Percent	Response Count
Less than 3 months	10.7%	6
3-6 months	25.0%	14
6 months-1 year	23.2%	13
1-3 years	**33.9%**	19
More than 3 years	8.9%	5

4. Do you feel that you received or had access to adequate information to help you make your decision to have DBS?

	Response Percent	Response Count
Yes	**67.3%**	37
No	18.2%	10
Prefer not to answer	3.6%	2
Unsure	10.9%	6

5. Did you choose to have the surgery on your own, because you felt you needed to do it, or were you urged to do it by a care partner/family member/employer?

	Response Percent	Response Count
My doctor recommended it.	38.8%	19
I did it for myself	**65.3%**	32
I did it because someone else wanted me to	6.1%	3
I can't remember	0.0%	0
Prefer not to answer	0.0%	0

6. If you waited one year or more to have the surgery, what were your reasons? (You may check more than one answer. If you waited less than one year, skip this question.)

	Response Percent	Response Count
Symptoms "not bad enough yet"	**40.9%**	9
Hadn't tried all possible medications yet	18.2%	4
Too scared of the idea to really think about it	**40.9%**	9
Insurance/Medicare wouldn't pay	18.2%	4
Partner/family didn't like the idea	4.6%	1
Wanted to "shop around" to find the best surgeon/hospital	22.7%	5

7. If you had to make the decision over again, would you have the procedures done sooner?

	Response Percent	Response Count
Yes	**60.0%**	33
No	30.9%	17
Don't know	9.1%	5

8. What year did you have your DBS system implanted? (If you have had multiple surgeries, please list all years)

	Response Percent	Response Count
Before 2001	5.5%	3
2001	9.1%	5
2002	12.7%	7
2003	5.5%	3
2004	23.6%	13
2005	16.4%	9
2006	**27.3%**	15
2007	16.4%	9

9. How did you decide where to have your DBS done?

	Response Percent	Response Count
My doctor recommended a surgeon/facility.	**63.0%**	34
I chose the surgeon/facility closest to my home.	7.4%	4
I chose the least expensive surgeon/facility near me.	0.0%	0
I went to the surgeon/facility that my insurance covered.	5.6%	3
A surgeon/facility was recommended by someone else with PD.	9.3%	5
I did extensive research and then made my choice	13.0%	7

140

10. Who first recommended that you be evaluated for DBS?

	Response Percent	Response Count
My family doctor	0.0%	0
My neurologist	**60.0%**	33
A movement disorder specialist	32.7%	18
Another neurologist (second opinion)	3.6%	2
Don't remember	3.6%	2

11. Have you had DBS implanted on both sides (bilateral) or just one side (unilateral)? Do you have one neurostimulator/pacemaker or two?

	Response Percent	Response Count
One side, with one neurostimulator	12.7%	7
Both Sides, with one neurostimulator	41.8%	23
Both sides, with two neurostimulators	**43.6%**	24

12. Did you have any pain related to any of the surgeries (brain surgery or chest surgery)?

	Response Percent	Response Count
Yes, pain during surgery	5.7%	3
Yes, pain after surgery	**47.2%**	25
No, no pain	45.3%	24
Don't remember	0.0%	0

13. How many nights did you spend in the hospital (for all surgeries) combined)?

	Response Percent	Response Count
None	0.0%	0
1-2	**60.0%**	33
3-5	25.5%	14
5+	12.7%	7

14. Did you experience any complications during or shortly after surgery?

	Response Percent	Response Count
No	**73.2%**	41
Yes -- infection	10.7%	6
Yes -- bleeding/stroke	1.8%	1
Don't remember/would rather not say	0.0%	0

15. Do you feel that you were given or had access to adequate information to prepare you for surgery?

	Response Percent	Response Count
Yes	**65.5%**	36
No	25.5%	14

16. If you have experienced any hardware-related complications since the surgery, such as a broken wire, neurostimulator broke through the skin, etc., please describe them here. If not, leave blank.

	Response Count
answered question	14

17. Have you experienced any side effects since the surgery or has your care partner noticed anything? Check all that apply.

	Response Percent	Response Count
No side effects	13.0%	7
Slurred/garbled speech	38.9%	21
Softer voice	**55.6%**	30
Symptoms are worse	7.4%	4
Dyskinesia	20.4%	11
Balance is worse	37.0%	20
Tingling sensation	18.5%	10
Numbness	3.7%	2
Dizziness or light-headedness	18.5%	10
Worsening of coordination/movement problems	24.1%	13
Depression (that you didn't have before, or worsening of previous condition)	14.8%	8
Anxiety (that you didn't have before, or worsening of previous condition)	9.3%	5
Obsessive-compulsive behavior, such as gambling, shopping, sorting things	5.6%	3
Problems with sleep (that you didn't have before, or worsening of previous condition)	11.1%	6

18. How many programming sessions were required to find your best setting?

	Response Percent	Response Count
No programming done yet	1.8%	1
Haven't found best setting yet	14.3%	8
One	3.6%	2
Two	10.7%	6
Three	8.9%	5
Four	10.7%	6
Five	5.4%	3
More than five (list)	17.9%	10
Other (please specify)	**25.0%**	14

19. How many "maintenance" programming visits do you have each year, on average?

	Response Percent	Response Count
None	18.0%	9
1	8.0%	4
2	**22.0%**	**11**
3	16.0%	8
4	20.0%	10
5	0.0%	0
6	2.0%	1
More than 6	14.0%	7

20. How have the results of your DBS been, compared to your pre-surgery expectations?

	Response Percent	Response Count
Better than I expected	**58.5%**	31
About the same as I expected	15.1%	8
Worse than I expected	15.1%	8
Not better or worse, but different than I expected	9.4%	5
No change	0.0%	0
Unsure	0.0%	0

21. How does your care partner/family feel about the results, compared to their pre-surgery expectations? (If single, check "Does not apply")

	Response Percent	Response Count
Results were better than they expected	**52.8%**	28
Results were about the same as they expected	7.6%	4
Results were worse than they expected	17.0%	9
Results were different than they expected	7.6%	4
Unsure	3.8%	2
Does not apply	9.4%	5

145

22. Since you've had DBS, do you ever feel that your care partner, family or friends expect too much of you? (For example, expect you to do more chores or more work than you think you can handle)

	Response Percent	Response Count
Yes	27.8%	15
No	**64.8%**	35
Unsure	7.4%	4

23. Knowing what you know now, would you do it (DBS) all over again?

	Response Percent	Response Count
Yes	**83.9%**	47
No	5.4%	3
Unsure	10.7%	6

24. Do you have any suggestions for someone who is thinking about having DBS?

	Response Count
answered question	**50**

25. Geographical info:

Response Count

100.0%   58

State/Province:

State/Province	Count
AK	1
CA	7
DE	1
FL	2
GA	1
IA	1
KS	1
MA	2
MN	6
MS	1
MT	1
NC	4
NE	2
NM	1
NV	1
OH	2
OR	2
PA	2

TX	8
VA	5
VT	1
WA	2
WI	4
Total:	58

Country: USA

26. About you:

	Response Percent	Response Count
male	**52.6%**	30
female	47.4%	27
	answered question	58
		100.0%

27. If you would like to be acknowledged in the book, please list your name, as you would like it printed (such as "Jackie C." "Jackie Christensen," etc.) If you want to be contacted about book publication, please list your email.

	Response Count
answered question	43

28. If you have questions or comments about the survey, please write them here. Or if you'd like to share more of your story, this is the place for it.

	Response Count
answered question	25

Acknowledgements

This book has been a long time coming! I owe a huge debt of gratitude to Sierra Farris, PA-C. She was the one who first planted the idea in my head in October 2005, just as my first book was being published. Now, three years later, I am finally finishing it, so my first words of appreciation go to Sierra! Thanks for the idea; the excellent programming sessions that have allowed me to function; your help with the electrophysiology chapter and review of the whole book; and your generosity with both your time and your expertise.

To my wonderful husband, Paul, who has seen me through so many things over the past twenty years, I love you truly, madly, deeply, infinitely.

Alex and Bennett, you are becoming gentle men like your father, before my very eyes! I am so glad that this technology has allowed me to be an active participant in your lives, and I thank you for all of your love and support as we have adjusted to living with my battery-operated brain.

Mom, thanks for your love and care, for coming to Cleveland in the dead of winter to see me through the brain surgery and for programming, and for helping to start the PD support group in Jackson.

Dad, thanks for your love and for sharing Mom. I only wish you could have lived long enough to see this!

Jack and Marge, I am so grateful for your support of all kinds throughout this process.

Kari Huseth, I don't know what we would have done without your assertiveness, your medical training, and your "lead foot" to get us back from Cleveland.

Annie Shull, thanks for taking time away from your understanding husband, Scott, and the wine biz so that Alex and Bennett could hang out with their Auntie Annie. Being with you instead of baby-sitters made them much more comfortable and less anxious about having both Paul and me away.

Kathy Hiltsley, you were invaluable as coordinator of meals during the surgery and have been a terrific friend!

The neuro team at Cleveland Clinic was amazing! I am forever indebted to Ali Rezai, MD; Scott Cooper, MD; Andre Machado, MD, PhD;

Cynthia Kubu, PhD; Monique Giroux, MD; Ellen Dooling, RN; Sierra Farris, PA-C; the staff; and anyone I may have missed at the Center for Neurological Restoration.

A big thank you to Paul Tuite, MD; Aviva Abosch, MD; Maggie Biebler, RN; and Susan Torgerson, RN; at the University of Minnesota, for serving as my local "pit crew." Dr. Tuite, I really appreciate your support and guidance these past ten years.

Thanks to Michael Okun, MD, for sharing the FLASQ-PD.

Carol Walton, your encouragement and editorial suggestions have been invaluable. The PD community is so lucky to have you and The Parkinson Alliance watching out for us.

Grazie to Bill Bell for being there for Paul and for me during and after the surgeries. The ice-bag tip was a lifesaver!

Last but far from least, I am tremendously grateful to all of the people living with PD who have shared their experiences and knowledge: Dr. Dave Heydrick; Gretchen and Michael; Gary and Maryanne; Jack and Judy; Bob and Susan; Andy and Deb; Gene; Vic and Carolyn; Connie; Steve; Roger; Magda; Ruth Hamilton; Vern Cork; Cheryl Cayo; Arthur E. Clough; Gupta Pandarinath, MD; Alice M. Crooker; Gary Mortensen; Kathy Greis; Steve Blostin; Char; Peter Torres; John K. Hanks; Deb W.; Richard J. Duell; Zenobia Sutton; Mike J.; Mike H.; Carol B. Meenen; Tricia L.; Ken Beebe; Alice G. Gross; Jerrold R. Wildenauer, DC; Michael Z.; Mary S.; Diabne Martinka; Garth Wilhem; W. Glenn Howells, PhD; Patricia Turley; Steve Heater; and anyone whom I may have forgotten.